The
Invisible
Orientation

THE
INVISIBLE
ORIENTATION

AN INTRODUCTION TO ASEXUALITY

JULIE SONDRA DECKER

CARREL BOOKS

Library of Congress Cataloging-in-Publication Data is available on file.

Cover design by Mary Belibasakis

ISBN: 978-1-63144-002-1
Ebook ISBN: 978-1-63144-017-5
Printed in the United States of America

TABLE OF CONTENTS

PART SIX: OTHER RESOURCES

ACKNOWLEDGMENTS

I would like to thank the following readers for their in-depth commentary, excellent analysis, and assistance in preparing this book:

Laura Sharp, Joseph Dante, Shawne Keevan, Helene Thompson, Hannah Hussey, Jessie Mannisto, Cristina C., Rebecca, and Laura.

Thanks go to the following readers for offering reactions, personal reflections, networking opportunities, support, and advice on the book:

Lydia White, Rachel Ward, Chandy Dancey, Marisa Kierra, Matthew Renetzky, Marisa Bishop, Aydan Selby, Lindsey Hampton, Brianne Nurse, Simon Parsons, Kristina Sanchez, Zanna Cooke, Jiselle Crawford, Sarah Sinnaeve, Kennedy St. John, Andrew Hinderliter, Emma Leslie, Kyle Evans, Patricia Wada, Charlie Glickman, David Jay, SL Huang, Whitney Fletcher, Emma MM, Eva, Nina, Christo, Amanda, Amy, Zoe, Ngina, Andreanne, Gabriel, Sarah, K.W., and Blow Pop.

For tolerating and supporting my sometimes obnoxious writerly habits and providing no shortage of unconditional love, immense thanks go to my parents, Marcia and Marlon, and my sisters, Patricia and Lindsay. Thank you also to my grandparents, my aunt, my brother-in-law, and all my honorary family. I give you all my eternal gratitude for all the support you've offered me on this journey.

For listening patiently to my tales of woe throughout the years and offering friendship with no strings attached, my heartfelt appreciation goes to these folks: Meghan, Jeaux, Victor, Jessie, Cara, Fred, Mike, Stacy, Sarah, Ronni, and R.

Thank you to the following asexual-spectrum bloggers whose borrowed words allowed this book to present a broader, more diverse picture of asexual experience:

Andrew Hinderliter, Audacious Ace, Aydan Selby, Dallas Bryson, Fiish, Ily, Jo Qualmann, Kaz, Laura, M. LeClerc, Mary Kame Ginoza, Queenie, Rebecca, Sciatrix, Tom, Tristan Miller, and those couple anonymous folks who know who they are.

I thank my agent, Andrea Somberg, for believing this book would change lives and offering her guidance to help make that happen. And I thank my editor, Nicole Frail, and the team at Skyhorse and Carrel Books for seeing value in my message and transforming my collection of rambles into an honest-to-goodness book.

Thanks to the following readers for sharing their unique perspectives, thereby greatly enhancing the book's accuracy and authenticity:

Elica Vaz Teixeira Santos, Sara Beth Brooks, Rafaela F. Ferraz, Anuar A Lequerica, Adrienne Whisman, Zelda MacFarland, Amber Francis, Dallas Bryson, Ashley Pratt, Cassie Walker, Elaine Capshaw, Colleen Dolan, Elliece Ramsey, Mara Seaborne, Glen Ireland, Jenna Bruck, Jennifer Wodtke, Julia Brankley, Kato Murray, Kayla Rubano, Matthew Pena, Ozy Frantz, Paul Kriese, Pete Rude, Rafaela Stancic, Samantha Finley, Shelby Riffle, Sonia Berg, Tatiana Taylor, Terra Albert, Artemis Gyccken, Tracy Foote, J. Ruddock, Cynthia Marie, Haley Marcayla, Luka R.C., Essie C, Gia S, Elliot T., Lou, Annie, Brittany, Amelia, Ellen, Lillia, Tas, Kai, Shayla, Blythe, Tom, H.X., Alicorn, Sciatrix, knittedace, Liara-shadowsong, The Scrabbler, nervous_neuron, ridiculousprocrastinator, singinglupines, iamdeltas, Infinite Tree, Asexual-poetry, The One in Purple, and Citation, Queen of Gibberish.

I couldn't have written this book without the support of my community. Thank you all.

INTRODUCTION

My Story

"It's not you, it's me."

At age fourteen, I had my first boyfriend. I wasn't attracted to him, but I kissed him a few times anyway because I was expected to. It certainly wasn't the thrilling experience movies and romance books had led me to expect. In fact, I could barely think of an experience I'd enjoyed less. But whenever I told people I thought so, they'd say, "You're fourteen. One day you'll like it."

At age sixteen, I left my second boyfriend perplexed and frustrated. I liked him as a person, but I wasn't interested in him the way he wanted me to be: definitely not sexually, and not even romantically. My disinterest in having sex with him wasn't rooted in the usual reasons—that "a lady" was expected to save herself, that I was afraid of sex, that I didn't want to get diseases or get pregnant—I simply had a complete lack of interest in sex and anything related. I didn't think sex was a gross concept. I didn't think it was immoral. I'd just never been sexually attracted to another person. Not my boyfriend, not the hottest people in school, not the heartthrob movie stars. I wasn't interested. Period.

My boyfriend dubbed me "Miss Non-Hormone." I called myself "nonsexual." I was reasonably sure that I would recognize sexual attraction if I felt it, but the mantra of "you can't know until you try it" did inspire me to experiment a bit. And all my experiences were exactly what I'd expected: at best tolerable, at worst uncomfortable. Never enjoyable, never exciting, never intriguing enough to make me want more. I broke up with the boy because he considered sex an essential element in a relationship, and I vowed to trust myself from then on as the authority on what I was feeling and what experiences I wanted. If this "sexual attraction" thing ever happened to me, I'd go with it, and if not, I had no reason to force it. At eighteen, I fully expected to develop a "normal" sexual appetite when I got older.

That was in 1996.

Nothing changed for me, and I made my peace with that, even though it was disorienting and sometimes alienating when nearly all my friends were either partnering up (and gleefully discussing the details) or acting depressed about their inability to do so.

The "concerned comments" began rolling in during my late teens and early twenties.

That's not normal. You need to get checked out.

You're never going to be happy.

I can fix you. I can help you.

You're a loser. You're a failure.

You have a disorder.

You're going to die alone with a houseful of cats.

Shut up and admit you're gay.

Why is it such a big deal to try sex?

You're selfish. You're a tease.

Women aren't supposed to like sex anyway.

You're trying to be different. You just want attention.

You're too ugly to get laid.

You're too pretty to go to waste.

Some of the people making these comments were well-meaning. Some of them found it offensive that sex didn't matter to me. Some felt my lack of interest in a central aspect of *their* lives somehow disrespected sex itself or the people who love it. And all of them wanted me to believe there was something wrong with me—and make me choose between fixing it and being properly ashamed of it.

But I was one of the lucky ones. I had a supportive family, unshakable confidence, no serious problems or issues in my life, and a thick skin. After encountering these attitudes again and again, I blew off some steam through writing an online essay about my experience as a nonsexual person in a sexual world, outlining both the negative reactions I regularly received and the reasons why I thought they were misguided. Sharing my story prompted a steady trickle of email from people who felt the same way—people who had fared far worse than I had.

It's isolating and lonely to be the only person around who lacks sexual attraction or interest in sex. I know this from experience, but I was used to defining and defending my feelings and choices through a privileged lens of high self-esteem. Without that core of confidence, the criticism I dealt with would have been nearly unbearable. Those dismissive messages are ubiquitous and incessant, and they can confuse and *hurt* people who don't have the kind of shield I had, leaving some unable to demand respect in their relationships and unable to connect with others who know what they're going through. And then those misleading and damaging messages take over their lives and become true, depriving them of the ability to have happy relationships of any kind. If everyone treats you like you're broken, you may eventually crack.

In the early 2000s, when I'd recently graduated from college, David Jay created the Asexual Visibility and Education Network (AVEN). David had been through many of the same experiences I had, and he had decided people like us needed resources and access to community. Many of the people I'd previously talked to found AVEN and developed a supportive network, shared their pride in their identity, and spearheaded the beginnings of outreach to educate the world about their orientation. When media outlets picked up on the concept, I started describing myself as "asexual" instead of "nonsexual" to connect myself with the awareness efforts, and I participated in some of the interview requests and took what opportunities I could to educate other people on the existence and experience of asexuality.

Having a network through which asexual people could find each other—along with a widespread acknowledgment that the orientation exists—was a great step forward. But it remains a terribly underdiscussed topic, which leaves the door open for the next generation of asexual teenagers to go through life hearing the same messages I did, very likely to lose confidence in their ability to form interpersonal connections during their formative years. Asexual people's friends and family frequently confront their loved ones with these messages because they have no idea that asexuality is a sexual orientation. The despair I read about in some of those early emails still haunts me.

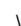 And now, I want to help other asexual people embrace their orientation without an instilled core of self-doubt. This will only become possible if everyone—asexual people and non-asexual people alike—can be given access to information about asexuality: what it is, what it isn't, who it affects, and why it doesn't need to be "cured."

What Is This Book About?

This book should function as a starting point for people interested in asexuality. It covers the basics of what asexuality is and isn't, explores the most common issues asexual people may be dealing with, presents some pointers for newly asexual-identified people and the people who love them, and includes some resources to find out more.

It is *not* meant to be taken as gospel. It is *not* meant to be a comprehensive look at the subject even though it covers a lot of ground. It is *not* a scientific or medical or psychological text—it's for the layperson, written in everyday language. It is *not* the final word on all-things-asexual, and though it is *not* just my personal story, it is *not* meant to be an attempt to speak for everyone.

It is, however, written to be a beginning.

Who Is This Book For?

This book is for people who are on the asexual spectrum, people who think they might be asexual, friends and family and partners of people who have come out as asexual, curious parties, and those looking for information on the subject for their school papers, sexuality studies, and alternative sexuality resources.

And it's for people who think asexuality doesn't exist.

Why Was This Book Written?

There should be a fairly concise language-accessible book on asexuality that anyone can find in their bookstores and libraries. Asexuality is more common than most people believe—currently estimated to describe 1 percent of the population[1] (and if that doesn't sound like much, consider that 1 percent of the population in the United States amounts to more than three million people). At the time of this writing, asexuality is mentioned in a handful of articles, on forums online, on the occasional somewhat sensationalistic television piece, and once in a while in documentaries and fictional works. There's not much information about it in mainstream publications. This conspicuous absence helps contribute to the overall perception that asexuality doesn't exist. After all, if something exists, shouldn't there be a book on it?

The average asexual person spends too many of their formative years hearing explicit and implicit negative messages about lack of sexual attraction or interest. It doesn't take much to severely warp an impressionable, still-forming young mind.

Asexual people are realizing they're asexual at the same time most other people start experiencing sexual attraction for the first time. It's scary to be left

---

1 One percent in a sample of eighteen thousand British adults agreed with the statement "I have never felt sexually attracted to anyone at all." (Bogaert, 2004)

out, and it's even scarier to be told that failure to experience this attraction indicates something terribly wrong.[2]

So asexual people sometimes feel they have to try to fit in, bury their true feelings, lie about their orientation, and go to great lengths to cover it up, privately terrified they're deeply flawed. They are led to believe through the media, through messages from their friends, and through pressure from interested partners that not feeling sexual attraction or not desiring others sexually is pathological. Asexuality needs to be in the common consciousness so asexual people across the board know their feelings have a name—and can stop thinking they're broken if they don't conform.

Some concerned sex experts say late bloomers might latch onto the "asexual" bandwagon if they know it's there and resist "blooming" when it happens to them.[3] However, it's important for the general population to realize asexuality is a possibility. Asexuality awareness doesn't become dangerous just because some people might mislabel themselves while they're still figuring out their feelings. *Lack* of awareness is certainly dangerous to asexual people, though.

Many asexual people who discover the orientation via the Internet have a massive relief response, pouring out their stories to faceless audiences, grateful to find they aren't alone. It's wonderful to find one's community, but the desperation that leads up to these reactions is the product of years of anxiety and fear. It's alienating to be marginalized so thoroughly, so completely—to think you can't connect with others in a way that most portray as necessary and natural for everyone—and many people deal with this rejection by rejecting and hating themselves.

Non-asexual people should know about asexuality so they can avoid perpetuating these messages and instead become supportive—as well as have good relationships with the asexual people in their lives—and asexual people should be able to explore their identities without facing prepackaged sexuality boxes that exclude them and deny their existence.

This book was written because everyone will benefit from knowing that asexuality exists, that it isn't a disorder, and that asexual people can be trusted to describe their own feelings—even if their answer for who they are sexually interested in is "none of the above."

---

2 "Coming to identify as asexual requires that individuals reject a widely-held cultural ideology of sexuality as biologically based and ubiquitous. [. . .] [T]hey draw attention to an oft overlooked social assumption—that all humans possess sexual desire." (Scherrer K., 2008)

3 "Just because someone is in her late teens or early twenties doesn't mean she is necessarily in full bloom. What you feel now may not be who you are so much as where you are in your own unique cycle of development. By labeling yourself too soon, you run a serious risk of mislabeling yourself, then feeling duty-bound to live up to it." Dr. Joy Davidson (ABC 20/20, 2006)

PART ONE:
ASEXUALITY 101

The Basics

ASEXUALITY IS:

Asexual orientation currently estimated to describe 1 percent of the population. Asexuality is usually defined as the experience of not being sexually attracted to others. Less commonly, it is defined as not valuing sex or sexual attraction enough to pursue it.

WE'RE NOT:

Asexuality isn't a complex. It's not a sickness. It's not an automatic sign of trauma. It's not a behavior. It's not the result of a decision. It's not a chastity vow or an expression that we're "saving ourselves." We aren't by definition religious. We aren't calling ourselves asexual as a statement of purity or moral superiority.

We're not amoebas or plants. We aren't automatically gender confused, anti-gay, anti-straight, anti-any-sexual-orientation, anti-woman, anti-man, anti-any-gender, or anti-sex. We aren't automatically going through a phase, following a trend, or trying to rebel. We aren't defined by prudishness. We aren't calling ourselves asexual because we failed to find a suitable partner. We aren't necessarily afraid of intimacy. And we aren't asking for anyone to "fix" us.

WE DON'T:

Asexual people don't all look down on sex or people who have sex. We don't all avoid romantic or emotionally close relationships, and we aren't automatically socially inept. We aren't defined by atypical biology or nonfunctional genitals. We aren't defined by mental illness, autism, or disability. We don't try to recruit anyone.

We don't have a hole in our lives where sexual attraction "should" be. We can't be converted by trying sex. We aren't, by definition, lonely or empty.

We aren't, by definition, immature or incompetent. We aren't, as a group, uglier or prettier than anyone else. We don't tell people not to have sex in the name of our orientation, nor do we use the term *asexual* to imply perceiving ourselves to be "above" sex.

WE SOMETIMES:

Some want romance. Some don't. Some are willing to have sex. Some aren't. Some are virgins. Some aren't. Some masturbate, or have a libido, or want children. Some don't. Some feel isolated, afraid, confused, othered, erased, and invisible. We wish we didn't.

SO PLEASE:

If you're not asexual, listen to us. Trust us to describe our own feelings. Understand that happiness isn't defined by traditional sexual relationships. Don't assume we need therapy or treat us like we need to be cured or tell us we're broken. Our rarity forces many of us to go through life without the understanding and support of others like ourselves. We want to be understood outside the deliberately constructed communities in which we're talking to ourselves, and that's why we need you. We want to combat the negative messages that make us feel invisible. If we're introducing you to asexuality, that means we're inviting you to understand.

Meet us halfway.

Asexuality Is a Sexual Orientation

What does it mean to identify as asexual?

If someone says "I'm asexual," usually they're expressing that they aren't sexually attracted to other people.[1]

ASEXUALITY: A sexual orientation characterized by sexual attraction to no one. Approximately 1 in 100 people is asexual.

In some cases, people who identify as asexual are expressing that, for them, sex isn't intrinsically worth pursuing for its own sake, or that they aren't interested in sex, or that they don't want or don't enjoy sex, or that they don't want to make sex part of their relationships. But regardless

---

1 "An asexual is someone who does not experience sexual attraction." (Asexual Visibility and Education Network, 2008)

of what definition someone uses, asexuality as a **sexual orientation** should be respected. Some asexual people prefer to see asexuality as a lack of sexual orientation, which is also a valid interpretation, but many prefer to say that their sexual orientation is, simply, attraction to no one.

Most people use the term *sexual orientation* as shorthand for "what kinds of people are sexy to me." But when asexual people answer that question with "no one, thank you," some non-asexual people resist processing that answer. Our society is used to hearing breakdowns: heterosexuality means experiencing cross-sex or cross-gender attraction, and everyone else is gay, bi, or pansexual. But when someone answers the "Who's sexy?" question with a blank, the world often yells "Hey, that's impossible!"[2]

This interpretation constitutes an unnecessarily black-and-white understanding of attraction. Even within the more popular orientations, it's not always simple. **For *everyone*, sexual orientation is more like a range, not a simple series of separate categories.** (Especially since gender isn't as simple as "male or female/man or woman," which complicates how we describe what genders we're attracted to; some people are between, outside, or a mixture of the binary genders.[3])

Describing attraction can get very complex, but for an asexual person, sexual attraction or inclination is toward "no one." That's not the same as not having developed a sexual orientation *yet*. Asexuality may look like a blank space waiting to be filled, but even if an asexual person never changes, their orientation is indistinguishable from "not yet" on the outside. It's impossible to prove a negative.

So if asexuality looks like a big nothing, how is that different from not having a sexual orientation at all? Some say the difference is analogous to a situation that can occur on a multiple-choice test. If answer choice D allows the test-taker to say "none of the above," that's very different from simply not answering the question. It's certainly going to be graded differently. Asexuality *is* an answer to the question, even if that answer is "none." It's not just a shrug. The word *none* can still fill in a blank.

---

2 "To concede that there are two forms of desire—cross-sex and same-sex desire—is to recognize the analytic possibility of at least four kinds of persons. These include: (1) those who harbor cross-sex but not same-sex desire; (2) those who harbor same-sex but not cross-sex desire; (3) those who harbor both forms of desire; and (4) those who harbor neither form of desire. Yet even those who acknowledge that orientation arrays itself on a continuum spanning the first three categories often ignore the fact that the continuum fails to represent the fourth." (Yoshino, 2000)

3 "Our internal sense of gender relates to our feelings of being a man, a woman, some combination, or neither. Traditionally it was believed that if you felt masculine you would not feel feminine, and vice versa. But [. . .] some people feel differing degrees of masculinity and differing degrees of femininity. Some people do not feel particularly like a man or a woman, and some feel that they have qualities of both." (Girshick, 2008)

> "I've known for years that I'm not like other people when it comes to sex, but I always just thought I was simply not very good at being straight."
>
> —TOM, ASEXUALITY ARCHIVE

Asexual people can say they *haven't* experienced sexual attraction, but yes, it's true they can't be sure it couldn't happen, logically speaking. However, they *can* be about as sure as anyone else about who they are attracted to, even if it happens to be no one. After all, people who are only attracted to one sex or gender aren't generally interpreted as "not yet" bisexual, but asexual people are held to a different standard.

The past and the present are usually good predictors of the future. Most people identify their orientation based on past and present attractions, so it naturally follows that asexual people could do the same and still have their orientation respected.

When a person has no sexual attraction to others or doesn't seek out sex, some may view that person as an undeveloped heterosexual person, as though being straight is the default. **But sexual orientation is not determined by whether someone has sex or who they have it with. Orientation is not a behavior—not for asexual people and not for anyone.** People who are sexually attracted to cross-gender partners are still heterosexual even if they have not had sex with a cross-gender partner. No one suggests heterosexual teenagers should identify as asexual until such time as they become heterosexual through sex with a cross-gender partner. Abstaining from sex is not the same thing as asexuality; it is the experience of attraction, not the behavior, which defines a person's orientation.

With 1 in 100 people not experiencing sexual attraction and/or not feeling motivated by or interested in sex, that's a lot of people wandering around largely unacknowledged. The 1-percent figure came from a large survey of eighteen thousand people administered in Britain, with 1 in every 100 people surveyed agreeing with the statement "I have never felt sexually attracted to anyone."

Some say this figure could be an overestimation because some technicalities could allow people who are not asexual to agree with that statement. And some say it is an underestimation, since some of the 99 percent may not know how to define sexual attraction and assume they have felt it even if they haven't. Some people misinterpret aesthetic appreciation, romantic attraction, or sexual arousal as being sexual attraction, only to realize later that they are asexual. Since this initial sample, researcher Anthony Bogaert has continued to study asexual people, and says the other samples he's reviewed up until the present suggest this figure is still somewhat accurate.[4]

That said, asexual communities are growing as awareness spreads, with more and more people recognizing themselves in the definitions every day. Respecting their orientation is important regardless of the numbers.

Asexuality Is a Mature State

Just like some people can't see the difference between "an asexual orientation" and "no orientation," many also can't see why "not interested" isn't the same as "not interested *yet*." Asexuality describes a mature state, not a passing phase or a blank spot before "real" maturation. *Asexual* isn't something you call a child before they reach sexual maturity. Asexuality applies to maturing or mature people.

Asexual people are often told they will one day find "the one" and develop sexual feelings and the values society attaches to them. Many asexual folks have to hear this over and over

> "I always laugh when I see these claims. I'm thirty-nine years old. It stopped being plausible a very long time ago that I could just be a 'late bloomer.' Yes, there are asexuals in their thirties. We exist. Our asexuality exists."
> —LAURA, *NOTES OF AN ASEXUAL MUSLIM*

and over again, which thrusts a perpetual image of immaturity upon them. Asexuality is not a signal that a person is necessarily stunted emotionally or physically, and feeling sexual attraction or inclination is not the line everyone must cross to be treated like an adult. Maturity should not be measured by willingness or inclination to seek out or accept sexual experiences.

Maturity doesn't have a specific definition with check boxes to tick off. It's common for people—especially people who are in few or no marginalized groups—to define maturity, functionality, happiness, and normality against their own standards, which they present as universal. Because of this, it's common for people who consider sex and sexual attraction part of their adult lives to say, "If you don't have sexual interest, you don't have an adult life."

Asexuality challenges this . . . and it should. **Plenty of people who desire or engage in sex are immature. It doesn't make sense to insist that someone must be immature if they don't have or desire sex.** Maturity is subjective,

---

4 "There's been other more recent kinds of well-conducted studies and they've varied in terms of the type of question that they asked, along with the percentages that they give, and I think still about a reasonable ballpark figure, at least in my mind, after reviewing some of that work is that 1 percent is probably not a bad figure, a sort of working figure." Anthony Bogaert on the *Colin McEnroe Show* (Bogaert A., 2013)

and how/when it manifests is highly individual. Asexual people usually develop mature adult lives and relationships just fine. The huge amount of diversity in how adults find success and happiness should be acknowledged, even if some adults don't seek out certain types of partnerships or certain kinds of intimate experiences.

Asexuality Is a Description

A sexual orientation is not a decision. A person's sexual orientation *describes* how that person experiences attraction.

It does not describe any decision that person makes about expressing sexuality, and it does not represent a vow or an intention regarding sex. Much like a heterosexual person does not "decide" when to start being attracted to partners, an asexual person doesn't "decide" no one is sexually attractive or worth pursuing sexually. It just happens.

Asexual people are often asked why, how, or when they "decided" to be asexual—usually by a well-meaning person who believes orientation can be chosen. People who ask this question generally feel asexual people are shutting themselves off from something wonderful—something they themselves find satisfying and fulfilling—and they can't understand why an asexual person would "choose" to forgo such experiences.

Sometimes it helps if these people can understand that it wasn't a choice, and that for the asexual person, engaging in sex might not be the fulfilling experience that it is for them. Asexual people can—and often do—decide to have sex. After all, people of any orientation *can* have sex with partners to whom they are not attracted. **But asexuality is about attraction, not about willingness to engage in sexual behavior.**

If someone who has never been sexually attracted to anyone does develop a sexual attraction, that person may decide to start using a different label. Labels are chosen to describe people—to be able to discuss the issues, find similar people, and understand the experience. When circumstances change, labels can too. There's no danger in asexual people describing themselves as asexual because it is not a decision they're now sworn to adhere to.

If someone's hair color or weight or marital status changes, they change how they describe themselves. **The change in description does not mean they weren't an authentic example of what the previous label described when it fit them.** For some people, sexual orientation is fluid.[5] So there's no

---

5 Lisa M. Diamond defines sexual fluidity as situation-dependent flexibility in sexual responsiveness. (Diamond, 2008)

need for anyone to fear that identifying as asexual might become a regrettable mistake. If it changes or turns out to be inaccurate, the asexual person can drop the label. It is not a chastity vow. Asexual communities have a happy history of supporting people who grow to understand that they are not asexual, just like they support those who continue to identify that way.

Asexuality Is a Healthy Status

"But sex is natural!"

Sex is commonly upheld as a normal and necessary part of all people's lives—especially if it's heterosexual, potentially procreative sex. The association between heterosexual sex and procreation is sometimes used as an excuse to invalidate other types of sex, though many forms of non-procreative sex are also dubbed "natural" by the majority. But then asexual people come along, describing a lack of sexual attraction or a lack of interest in sex, and all of a sudden the word *unnatural* rings out.

Peculiarly, those who invoke presumed avoidance of procreation as proof that asexual people are unnatural won't often use that argument to invalidate heteronormative, sexually active, but non-procreative lifestyles. It's very rare to hear "that's unnatural!" applied to heterosexual cisgender[6] people who use non-procreative sex positions, have sex using birth control, or have sex that involves a postmenopausal or otherwise infertile partner, even though procreation cannot result from these couplings. This is because labeling asexuality as unnatural is not actually about reproduction, even when detractors claim it is. It's about intimate connection—and about the misconception that asexual people cannot experience a supposedly necessary connection with others unless they have sex. Asexual people often cannot be recognized as whole or healthy people if they lack sex, sexual attraction, or sexual inclination in their lives.

Most asexual people can have procreative sex if they wish to; they just happen to have inclinations that are less likely to lead to procreative sex. Even if they have had children or plan to, they will *still* hear their desires described as unnatural. If someone doesn't want a connection through sex, that's when the in-depth personal questions about medical history begin. Yes, it is possible to have a hormone deficiency,[7] or an illness,[8] or to be on a medication that contributes to lack

---

6 "Cisgender" or "cis" refers to those whose gender matches the sex they were assigned or designated at birth, distinguishing them from people who *don't* identify as the gender they were assigned/designated.

7 "[M]inimal critical levels of androgens appear necessary (although not sufficient) for the experience of sexual desire." (Regan, 1999)

8 "Medical conditions are a frequent source of direct or indirect sexual difficulties. Vascular disease associated with diabetes might preclude adequate arousal; cardiovascular disease may inhibit intercourse secondary to dyspnea." (Phillips, 2000)

of interest in or enjoyment of sex.[9] In nearly all cases there are other primary effects besides those relating to sex or arousal, though, especially in the case of atypical hormones; lack of sexual interest can be a symptom of a broader condition, but it is *not* an illness in and of itself. Despite that, "you'd better get your hormones checked" is one of the most common reactions asexual people hear.

Yes, getting tested for abnormalities and paying attention to health are very good habits to form. But there is no evidence that asexual people's hormones are produced differently from anyone else's. However, it has been noted that asexual people sometimes have a higher incidence of late and less dramatic puberty,[10] though plenty of people with the exact opposite situation also identify as asexual.

When discussing hormones, it's relevant to mention that some asexual people have lowered or absent production of certain hormones, and it is not necessarily "to blame" for their orientation just because hormones are linked to puberty and sex. This becomes particularly relevant in discussing populations known to have atypical hormone production, like those with certain intersex variations.[11] (*Intersex* refers to people who are born with chromosomes or anatomy/physiology that is not exclusively considered typically male or female.) Some intersex individuals identify as asexual,[12] but their sexual orientation shouldn't be assumed to be a "symptom" of their intersex variation that needs fixing. Some who use medication to control or change their hormones still identify as asexual.

In most cases, lack of sexual interest or attraction is unlikely to be caused by any physical issue, hormonal or otherwise. Asexuality also isn't enough to indicate a psychological problem. If a person's sexual interest was present and then disappeared suddenly, that might be a physical or psychological issue.[13] If a person feels that trauma is getting in the way of going through with desired sexual interactions, that person can choose to pursue counseling.

---

9 "Many commonly used drugs can interfere with sexual function in both men and women, causing loss of libido, interfering with erection or ejaculation in men, and delaying or preventing orgasm in women." (Medical Letter on Drugs and Therapeutics, 1992)

10 "[A]sexual women had a later onset of menarche relative to the sexual women. Asexual people were also shorter and weighed less than the sexual people." (Bogaert, 2004)

11 "[I]n [intersex] conditions with gonadal dysgenesis where the gonads are non-functioning there is no endogenous hormone production. . . ." (Minto, Crouch, Conway & Creighton, 2005)

12 In a survey of 3,436 self-identified asexual-spectrum people administered on the Internet in September–October 2011, 1.2 percent identified themselves as intersex (Asexual Awareness Week, 2011). That percentage is comparable to the percentage of intersex individuals in the overall human population.

13 "[A] decrease in sexual desire can signal psychological or physiological disorders (e.g., depression, hypothyroidism), but is low or absent sexual desire necessarily associated with pathology? [. . .] Currently, evidence does not suggest that cognitions and behaviors associated with asexuality necessarily signal a problem." (Prause & Graham, 2007)

If sexual appetite, sex drive, or sexual interest has declined because of medication and the patient is distressed by this, alternative therapies can be discussed and possibly applied.[14]

It is of course possible for a person to be mentally and/or physically ill *and* asexual without either of those traits being blamed for the other. Even if a physical or mental disease is part of a person's overall reason for feeling asexual, that does not invalidate the orientation for that person; it does not become less "real" because of any illness. **However, asexuality as an orientation is not a disease or a symptom. It shouldn't be treated like an issue that can or should be cured,** any more than homosexuality should.

> "I think a search for a cause for one's asexuality can too often go down a road of biological determinism, which leads to questions of hormone levels or an asexuality gene. It devalues the role of the myriad other aspects of one's life in molding who one is as a person."
> —M. LeClerc, *Hypomnemata*

Asexuality is *especially* unlikely to be indicative of a detrimental condition if the asexual person in question is embracing it. Finding a name for one's experiences—and realizing that it isn't a sickness or a disorder or a hurdle to leap—is usually a self-affirming experience. For some non-asexual people, sexual attraction is such an integral part of life that they can't help but imagine an asexual life as depressing and fear-inspiring, so it's not surprising when some respond with concern while urging asexual people to get help. But if asexual people are relieved and happy to find they don't have to force themselves to "be sexual" to lead fulfilling lives, it's a lot more likely that trying to help by pushing them toward sexual experiences at all costs will be of no help at all.

Asexuality Is a Reasonable Possibility

Because lack of sexual interest or attraction is often medicalized or thought of as a disorder, it's very common for detractors to want "justification" from asexual people. In their minds, asexual people must prove their sexual orientation is not caused by something else in their lives before they will consider the possibility that the asexual person is really asexual.

---

14 "No medical treatment is available specific to patients with disorders of desire. If no underlying medical or hormonal etiology is discovered, individual or couple counseling may be helpful." (Phillips, 2000)

> "Asexuality isn't something diagnosed by a blood test or MRI scan. (. . .) Definition of asexuality is 'lack of sexual attraction,' another one I've seen and like is 'you're asexual if you think the label fits and is useful for you.' Neither of those are in any way something science can *confirm*. Both of those are something that each person knows for themselves."
>
> —KAZ, *KAZ'S TUMBLINGS*

Asexuality is not a last resort diagnosis. It is not a diagnosis at all. Studies on asexual people have not suggested a correlation with mental illness,[15] though some studies suggest asexual people who feel like outsiders in society can experience depression and other issues[16]—just like *anyone* who feels like an outsider is more susceptible to being depressed and anxious. Asexuality also doesn't refer to a physical inability to become aroused. There is no reason to search for "damning" evidence in asexual people's pasts, their medical history, their gender identity, their social status, their sexual experiences, their mental health, their physical attractiveness, their attitudes toward sex, or their age to conclude that someone isn't asexual (or that asexuality isn't real).

In asexual communities, there is a type of asexual person jokingly referred to as the *gold-star asexual*—an asexual person who lacks all the traits often blamed for asexuality, and therefore supposedly makes a good spokesperson since they are, for all intents and purposes, unassailable. Gold-star asexual people are not inherently better representations for asexuality, but they are frequently used to that effect, and this can spread unrealistic expectations and misunderstandings about the orientation.

Gold-star asexual people have the following traits:

- Are healthy (mentally and physically, not on medication)
- Are able-bodied
- Have never experienced abuse
- Are extroverted and/or socially competent
- Are cisgender (not transgender, non-binary, gender fluid, agender, genderqueer, neutrois, bigender, third gender, or gender questioning)
- Are supportive of others' consensual sex practices (though indifferent to sex themselves)
- Don't have a libido

---

15 "There were not higher rates of psychopathology among asexuals." (Brotto, Knudson, Inskip, Rhodes & Erskine, 2010)

16 "Because asexual individuals may face similar social stigma to that experienced by homosexual and bisexual persons, in that they may also experience discrimination and/or marginalisation, it follows that asexual individuals might also experience higher rates of psychiatric disturbance." (Yule, Brotto & Gorzalka, 2013)

- Are physically attractive
- Are not interested in romantic relationships (or, sometimes, are interested in hetero relationships)
- Are between the ages of twenty and forty

Of course, even asexual people in this "sweet spot" are often targeted with dismissive statements, but any asexual person who also lacks one or more of the above traits will often be immediately dismissed as "not really asexual" because of it.

Asexuality is more common than most people believe, and it only stands to reason that some percentage of the millions of asexual people would be, for instance, abuse survivors, mentally ill, normatively unattractive, gender nonconforming, or shy. It's not realistic to assign these traits the blame for those people's asexuality and only agree to "grant" belief in their orientation if all other possibilities have been eliminated.

To review: this chapter covered what asexuality is, as opposed to what it is not. Asexuality is a **sexual orientation** because it describes a person's pattern of attraction (to no one). Asexuality is a **mature state** because it isn't a term for what a person is before they develop their sexual orientation. Asexuality is a **description** because it is a word for explaining an experience, not a decision or a choice. Asexuality is a **healthy status** because it is not considered a mental or physical illness to not desire, pursue, or feel attraction that leads to sex. And it is a **reasonable possibility** because feeling sexual attraction or inclination toward others is not the default.

Asexual people shouldn't be obligated to undertake exhaustive attempts to embrace any other sexual orientation before they're allowed to "give up" and acknowledge that they're asexual. If a person hears the word and relates to one of the definitions, it very well may be the right label for them. The rest of this book should help paint a clearer picture of what asexual life looks like, what asexuality is not, and what both asexual and non-asexual people need to know about asexuality.

PART TWO:
ASEXUAL EXPERIENCES

The common thread all asexual people have is that they don't get sexually attracted to (or sexually inclined toward) other people. There are further subdivisions that describe the asexual experience in different ways, and sometimes they seem confusing outside asexual circles. All too often, asexual people hear "You can't be asexual if you masturbate!" or "You can't be asexual if you have a boyfriend!" or "What's the point of saying you're asexual if you have sex?" So this section should clarify how different types of asexual folks fit under the big asexual umbrella.

Romantic Orientation

One distinction between types of asexual people is whether they are romantically attracted to others or desire romantic relationships. Asexual people who are romantically attracted to others are called, predictably, **romantic asexual** people.

Romanticism

Relationships do not have to include sex or sexual attraction to be categorized as romantic. Some asexual people do have the

"My romantic partner is also my best friend. I can't point out any specific thing that makes our relationship romantic, but it definitely is."
—REBECCA

desire for partnered relationships that cannot be described as "just friendship," though it's a common misconception that all asexual people lack the capacity for romantic love. The opposite situation—sex or sexual attraction between people who are not in love—is universally acknowledged. Sex can even be great between people who aren't in love! But love without sex (or the desire for it) is frequently called out as impossible, or at least unequal to "real" love.

We all understand, conceptually, that a positive emotion we call love can exist without sex or sexual attraction—familial love, friendly love, the deep and burning love for a good plate of mashed potatoes. But sometimes, **when a person**

describes a romantic relationship existing without the sexual element, suddenly that person's love is judged as puppy love, immature love, fairytale love, or something dysfunctional. People who love romantically without sexual attraction are often considered unqualified to describe their own feelings properly . . . as if the majority gets to be the authority on the minority's emotions. But desire for sex does not define desire for romance, any more than love's presence or absence defines whether sex happens.

Some asexual people, despite not feeling sexual attraction to their partners, nevertheless *do* want to have satisfying romantic relationships in which the partners can fulfill each other's needs. **People outside this equation do not get to say what feelings are possible for asexual people, nor do they define what needs must be mutually satisfied for the relationship to "count."** People who do experience sexual attraction can help spread understanding by acknowledging that no one is qualified to grant or deny legitimacy for another person's relationship. Asexual and non-asexual people can coexist and respect each other's way of life without making claims of exclusivity over whose relationships count.

Except for asexual people's lack of sexual attraction to those they love, all their other feelings can be as varied and intense as those of anyone else. Love and sex do happen to be intertwined for a great many people, and since these experiences bounce off one another to enhance and affect the overall experience, it's popularly believed that one is *necessary* for the other to work properly. This is not the case for everyone. Sex *can and does happen* without love and it is "real" sex, so why would love require sex to be desired or performed before it can be considered "real"?

> "For some asexual people, the thought 'I would like to have sex with that person' could seem as random and unexpected as 'I would like to paint that person blue, cover them with twigs, and dance around them in a circle all night.'"
> —TOM, *ASEXUALITY ARCHIVE*

For many asexual people, expressing feelings of love and closeness through sex just doesn't naturally occur to them, or sex doesn't seem like it is intrinsically attached to love. They may seem like separate experiences. Many romantic asexual people have a difficult time realizing they are asexual if they have romantic interests. They may think they can't be asexual because they still like people romantically, but don't think of their crushes in a sexual manner. It can be alienating when crushes don't follow the popular formula; many asexual adolescents even lie to their peers about finding people sexually attractive just to make their crushes sound more like their friends'.

For asexual people who experience it, romantic attraction is an independent experience from sexual attraction, which may look odd from an outside perspective. If it's real and intense and compelling, then why doesn't it inspire the feelings most people expect when they feel it themselves? Believing the love isn't fully there unless sex is desired too is like believing a tailless dog is never happy based on the notion that all dogs wag their tails if they're happy. For asexual people, sexual attraction is just not in the equation; like the tailless dog, it's just not there to wag. Romantic attraction without sexual attraction is the way a romantic asexual person operates. And it's every bit as compelling—and satisfying—when it happens.

Asexual people are the best judges of whether their relationships are romantic. **Most would say a relationship becomes romantic when its participants cross a**

> "We receive messages everywhere that tell us sex and romance go hand in hand, and I'm sure they do for some people. However, this becomes problematic when this experience is perceived as 'correct' or 'normal.'"
> —AUDACIOUS ACE, *ASEXUALITY UNABASHED*

certain threshold of intimacy and access to each other's lives. That threshold doesn't have to be sexual. People in romantic relationships include their partners in exclusive experiences and offer each other private knowledge, and that comfort and trust does not become possible only between people who are also being intimate sexually.

If relationship participants are having sex and they say they're in love, a knee-jerk response of "no you're not!" would be very rare indeed, not to mention rude. For relationship participants involving one or more asexual people, that same knee-jerk response is standard, and many people wouldn't consider it rude. Asexual people hear this type of invalidation all the time; they are frequently expected to defend their relationships' legitimacy and are regularly told their minds and hearts must not work right if their genitals don't get involved.

Sexual attraction is not the only drive that motivates partner selection. Some assume that if an asexual person has no sexual attraction to potential partners, that person would be able to be romantically attracted to any person regardless of sex, gender, gender expression, personality, aesthetic, or physical trait. That doesn't happen to be true. Aesthetic attraction exists, and some who experience no sexual attraction will still prefer partners they think are physically attractive. Many heterosexual people have a "type" of cross-gender partner they're attracted to; even if a heterosexual man would normally say he's attracted to "women," it might be true that he is primarily attracted to only a subsection of women. Asexual people often have a type as well, which is sometimes dependent on gender or gender presentation.[1]

Common Romantic Orientations	
Heteroromantic	Romantically attracted to cross-sex or cross-gender people
Homoromantic	Romantically attracted to same-sex or same-gender people
Biromantic or ambiromantic	Romantically attracted to more than one sex or gender.
Polyromantic	Romantically attracted to multiple sexes or genders but not *all* sexes and genders (note: this is not the same as being polyamorous)
Panromantic	Romantically attracted to people of all sexes and genders

For example, an **asexual heteroromantic** woman is not sexually attracted to anyone, but is romantically attracted to men. An **asexual polyromantic** man is not sexually attracted to anyone, but may be romantically attracted to women, agender people, and non-binary people, but not men (for example).

Also, some may see gender as more of a personality trait than a physical aesthetic, so attraction experiences can be less inclusive than "I'm attracted to X gender." Some may be attracted to those with a certain manifestation of femininity, masculinity, or androgyny or may prefer those who display a particular attitude when it appears within one gender but not within another (e.g., they may like aggressive women but not aggressive men or find graceful movements to be attractive in a man but have no reaction to similar gracefulness in a woman). Attraction is sometimes dependent on far more than a person's body or physical aesthetic.

Some people are also **unsure,** or **questioning,** or **fluid** in their romantic orientation. These romantic orientations are not restricted to asexual people; people who experience sexual attraction also have romantic orientations, and their romantic orientations may or may not correspond to their sexual attractions.

Asexual folks may use broader terms like *gay, straight,* or *queer* instead of *heteroromantic* and the like; you might encounter people identifying as *lesbian asexual* or other terms that are traditionally associated with assumedly sexual relationships. They are often referring to romantic orientation when they do this, though sometimes

---

1 "While a romantic dimension might be a relatively unique axis of sexuality, asexual individuals in this survey also described their sexual identity in relation to the gender of their partner(s). [. . .] None of the self identified aromantic asexual individuals [out of 11] indicated gender as important in relationships, in contrast to those who identify as romantic, where all but one [out of 22] described the gender of their partner(s) as important to their sexual identity." (Scherrer K., 2008)

they're defining themselves as such based on the gender of a non-romantic partner. (Non-romantic partner relationships will be discussed shortly.)

However, romantic attraction is not always simple considering there are more than two genders. Many people identify as non-binary genders; they don't fit in male or female boxes. They may identify as a mixture of both, or as shifting between genders, having no gender, or having a neutral gender. Those who don't identify as women or as men may use terms like *agender, gender neutral, neutrois, bi-gender, androgynous, non-binary, genderqueer, gender variant, gender fluid, gender questioning, without gender,* or *third gender.* (These will not be discussed in detail in this book, but it should be noted that some asexual people also have one of these non-binary gender identities.) As you might imagine, non-binary people may find the above romantic orientation terms especially unhelpful or inaccurate.

Instead of describing romantic attraction in terms of whether the desired partner is the same or different from one's own gender, some folks find it more useful to choose a term that describes their desired partner without describing themselves. While the more typical romantic orientations in the chart on the previous page are the ones you'll hear most in asexual communities, you may also see these (especially among non-binary or non-cisgender populations) to describe romantic attraction:

Additional Romantic Orientations	
Androromantic	Attracted to masculinity, men, or male-identifying/presenting people
Gyneromantic	Attracted to femininity, women, or female-identifying/presenting people
Skolioromantic or ambiromantic	Attracted to androgyny, non-binary, or androgynous-identifying/presenting people
Pomoromantic	Attracted to people, but do not consider it important to label or categorize their attractions (*pomo-* comes from *postmodern*)
Lithromantic	Attracted to people, but do not want that attraction reciprocated
Sapioromantic	Attracted to people based on intelligence

To be clear, people identifying as androromantic may be expressing that they are attracted to cis men *and* trans men and/or to masculinity and those who are masculine, while people identifying as gyneromantic may be expressing that they are attracted to cis women *and* trans women and/or to femininity and those who are feminine. And some might use these terms combined to express more specific attractions or broader attractions.

There is also a term for being attracted to transgender people, and that is **transromantic**. However, it is not a term that is to be used by cisgender people who are attracted to transgender people; only trans people who find themselves primarily attracted to other trans people may use this term. However, even within trans spaces, it's often considered problematic; it suggests an inability to feel attraction to someone unless they're trans, and while some trans people would rather only date someone else who's trans, that's not the same thing as who one finds attractive. Binary trans people generally expect and definitely deserve to be regarded as the gender they identify as, not an alternate version of that gender—meaning if someone is attracted to trans women, there's no need to specify beyond saying they're attracted to women. The term *transromantic* is very rarely used, but it does exist.

And finally, some asexual people are romantically attracted to one or more genders but do not pursue relationships because they believe the sexual needs are likely to be too mismatched and they don't believe it's worth the time and trouble to make it work.

But what about people who aren't attracted to anyone romantically?

Aromanticism

People who are not romantically attracted to others are called **aromantic**. They may stay single or pursue non-romantic partnerships of some kind; romantic partnerships aren't the only kind of committed relationship.

Aromantic folks are fairly common in asexual communities. While some romantic asexual people describe the interest in romance as a drive in and of itself—like a sex drive, a romantic drive can cause unattached people to wish for romantic partners and they may be romantically attracted to others—aromantic people don't experience this. People who identify as aromantic might describe themselves in one of the following ways:

- Having no romantic drive
- Not finding anyone attractive in a romantic sense
- Preferring singlehood
- Being satisfied by close friendships
- Not enjoying or relating to partnered life
- Feeling a general romantic interest ("I wish I had a partner, that would feel nice") but not actually finding anyone with whom they want a romance

Asexual people aren't the only orientation that can be aromantic; any sexual orientation might be romantically attracted to no one, and those who do pursue sexual relationships without romantic attraction are often shamed for it, so non-asexual aromantic folks face invisibility as well. Some people with perspectives along aromantic lines may prefer to identify as one of the gray areas of romantic orientation (discussed later in this chapter).

Many aromantic people grow up completely perplexed by what they are supposed to feel when their peers ask them, "So who do you like?" They may have been confused about how a crush was different from liking someone as a friend or may have felt compelled to make up crushes to avoid being left out, but just couldn't imagine what they'd want with a significant other. And as adults, they find that these partnerships are central to their peers' lives, and they may feel confused about how to pursue their futures without being constantly expected to want a mate. They may assume they want a romantic relationship because everyone suggests it's part of being happy, but then try dating and find they have nothing other than friendly feelings for their partners, leaving them in the dark as to what romance is supposed to feel like.

Some aromantic folks get all the social and emotional satisfaction they want from family and friendly relationships. Some simply have very little need for social or emotional interaction and would prefer to be alone most of the time. And then some have

> "When it comes to platonic relationships, we have . . . 'Friendship.' And that's really pretty much it. Sure, you can modify it: 'best friends,' 'childhood friends,' etc., but we still expect that one word to cover a huge spectrum of relationships. A 'friend' can refer to anything from someone you like to chat with a bit at lunch to someone you would like to spend the rest of your life with, would trust with your life."
> —MARY KAME GINOZA, *NEXT STEP: CAKE*

very close partnerships that seem closer than ordinary friendships, and they may include some aspects of physical and emotional intimacy and/or commitment, but there are differences in how they describe their partners if they have them. Aromantic relationships can include the following:

- A close relationship, but without a romantic relationship's *level* of access to each other's lives
- A close relationship, but without a romantic relationship's *type* of access to each other's lives
- A close relationship, but without a romantic relationship's *level* of closeness
- A close relationship, but without a romantic relationship's *type* of closeness
- A close relationship similar to romantic relationships in access and closeness, but does not seem romantic to the participants
- A close relationship that involves fulfilling participants' non-romantic needs

This does not imply that an aromantic partnership is necessarily less intense or less important than a romantic partnership—only that it is not what the members of the partnership define as romantic. What makes a relationship romantic is sometimes a heated discussion, but it becomes even more complicated when the prospects of sexual attraction and/or sexual encounters are removed from consideration.

"I don't particularly care who else someone I'm close friends with spends time with or whether they're dating someone. Exclusivity and monogamy are things I do not understand very well in a gut sense, and I don't really want either of them in any relationship for myself. That said—I recently walked away from a friendship with a person I cared very much about (and continue to care a lot about) because my emotional needs were not being met, largely because she didn't seem to think my company was worth seeking out. I do need to feel like a relationship has a similar level of affection on both ends to feel comfortable."

—Sciatrix, *Writing From Factor X*

Plenty of nonsexual and non-romantic types of attraction exist, including aesthetic, sensual, intellectual, and various kinds of emotional attraction. These can crop up independently of each other or in association with other kinds of attraction, and these elements can be intense, deep, and multifaceted. The prevailing cultural narrative tends to define all loving relationships as either sexual/romantic relationships, familial relationships, or friendships, but these distinctions are grossly oversimplified.

Friendships are often assumed less serious, less involved, and less important than any relationship that involves sex and/or romance. The word *just* appears in front of *friends* for that very reason. If people didn't believe sexual relationships automatically rank higher than nonsexual ones, the phrase *more than friends* wouldn't be so common. People wouldn't refer to friendships as arrangements in which "there's nothing between us." In reality, friendships can be among the deepest relationships people have—and that goes for everyone, not just aromantic people.

Some aromantic folks date—and that might sound like a contradiction, but **romance isn't the only type of serious and committed relationship a person might want to form**. Some seek devoted companions of a non-romantic type and may even want to raise children or cohabitate with a platonic partner. And many aromantic people don't have a partner even though they may have very close friendships. Some are perpetually single and happy that way.

The relationship descriptor **queerplatonic** gets a lot of mileage among aromantic asexual people, though anyone of any sexual or romantic orientation could have a queerplatonic relationship. Queerplatonic relationships are those that consist of dedicated, long-term partnership between the participants. The feelings between the partners are not romantic, but are still very powerful, and different in strength or type from what is usually reserved to describe typical friends.

The word *queerplatonic* is sometimes controversial because some say there is nothing "queer" about essentially having a best friend, but people in queerplatonic relationships may not feel comfortable describing their partnership as friendship, and their lifestyle is often mistaken for romantic from the outside. It is a platonic relationship, but it is "queered" in some way—not friends, not romantic partners, but something else. Sometimes these partnerships focus on the partners' shared goals or compatibility in areas of their lives not related to emotional attraction. A relationship shouldn't be assigned a romantic status if the participants say it is not romantic, even if it looks indistinguishable from romance when outside the equation.

Queerplatonic relationships tend to be misinterpreted as evidence of heterosexuality if they happen between cross-gender partners, and they tend to be misinterpreted as evidence of homosexuality if they happen between same-gender partners. But even if participants in a queerplatonic rela-

> "I tend to see the kinds of emotions I have as combining traits from both friendship and romantic models, which is why I usually use *queerplatonic relationship* and related terminology. I have listened to people describe relationships with similar levels of feeling to mine as either friendships or romantic relationships, and I really have a hard time figuring out where the distinction is. I also have a hard time figuring out where attraction comes into it, because for me it's a matter of strength of feeling, not type of feeling."
> —SCIATRIX, *WRITING FROM FACTOR X*

tionship want to live together permanently and even raise children or run a business or complete a goal together, that does not mean they are in a romantic relationship. It also does not tend to happen between most best-friend partnerships in Western society. It may be difficult for people who don't have close non-romantic relationships to understand if they happen to be content with the labels *friend* and *best friend* for their important non-familial/non-romantic relationships, but many people do feel this label describes something they previously did not have words for.

But is it possible to be somewhere in the middle here?

Grayromanticism
Gray areas of romantic experience exist, and there is terminology for those folks if they decide they want to label it. Some people describe themselves as

grayromantic—they're between romantic and aromantic. They experience romantic attraction much less often, to a lower degree, or under different circumstances than most people, having much in common with aromantic asexual people except that romantic attraction *does* happen for them once in a while. They may describe their grayromantic identity along with another one of the previously mentioned descriptors, such as *gray-panromantic* or *gray-androromantic*.

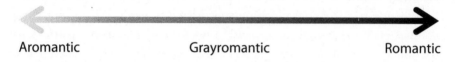

Aromantic   Grayromantic   Romantic

Demiromanticism

There are also **demiromantic** people. *Demiromantic* refers to a person who sometimes develops romantic attraction toward someone after becoming familiar with and emotionally fond of that person. Though some say that's how romance works for everyone, demiromantic people don't get crushes on strangers or people they don't know well—or they may describe it as never experiencing romantic attraction based on immediately apparent aspects of a person—and they may identify as demiromantic if it's very rare that they find someone romantically attractive.

These gray areas are not a uniquely asexual experience; grayromantic and demiromantic people may or may not experience *sexual* attraction in normative ways, but find their *romantic* experiences to be somewhere between aromantic and romantic. It's up to the gray-area folks to determine whether these terms are appropriate or useful for their relationships.

In a survey of 3,436 self-identified asexual-spectrum people administered on the Internet in September–October 2011, respondents answered "What is your romantic orientation?" in the following ways:[2]	
I am romantically attracted to **men**	43.8%
I am romantically attracted to **women**	32.2%
I am romantically attracted to **non-binary gender identified people**	21.1%
My romantic orientation is **fluid**	20.7%
I am **unsure** at this time	20.2%
I am romantically attracted to **no one (aromantic)**	18.2%
I am **demi-romantic**	12.1%

---

2 Community Census. (Asexual Awareness Week, 2011)

I am **gray-romantic**	10.6%
Other	6.8%
There is no difference between romantic and non romantic attraction to me	6.2%

* Participants were allowed to choose more than one answer.

Some people aren't sure how to describe their romantic orientation, or they reject the idea of specifically defining their attraction patterns, don't find any of the existing definitions useful in describing their feelings, or don't know whether they have a preferred gender or set of genders. A variety of creative ways exist to express this ambiguity. Terms that have been seen in asexual, aromantic, and questioning circles include **WTFromantic, quoiromantic, ambiguously romantic,** and **Schromantic** (describing romanticism in terms of Schrödinger's cat[3] as having the possibility of being romantic and aromantic at the same time).

To sum up, many asexual people experience nonsexual forms of attraction toward others. Asexual folks of all stripes should be able to use the phrase *significant other* without being told that their relationships are, for all intents and purposes, not significant enough. Aromantic asexual people should not be assumed to be single and looking or assumed resigned to single life due to failure to find a partner; many really enjoy being single and wouldn't have it any other way. Sexual orientation and romantic orientation are two different concepts.

Libido and Masturbation

Most openly asexual people are frequently asked to disclose explicit information about self-stimulation, often by strangers. Whether asexual people masturbate is a topic of much concern and curiosity.

The answer is that some asexual people do and some don't. Some have a sex drive and some don't. Some use toys and some don't. Some might even fantasize about certain experiences, while some don't.

If this sounds confusing, the main issue to remember is that sexual arousal, sex drive, and sexual attraction are different things.[4] *Sexual arousal* suggests a physiological response; *sex drive* suggests a desire to

---

3 Schrödinger's Cat is a thought experiment carried out by Erwin Schrödinger describing a cat put in a potentially lethal situation and hidden from the view of the experimenters, at which point they determined the cat, in quantum terms, is alive and dead at the same time.

4 "Asexuals reported significantly less desire for sex with a partner, lower sexual arousability, and lower sexual excitation but did not differ consistently from non-asexuals in their sexual inhibition scores or their desire to masturbate." (Prause & Graham, 2007)

respond to arousal or a desire to pursue sex; and *sexual attraction* suggests an experience of finding someone sexually appealing.

Asexual people are defined as asexual because other people aren't sexually attractive in their minds (or the possibility of sex with other people isn't particularly compelling). That does not mean that their genitals must be incapable of arousal; it does not mean they're necessarily unable to enjoy genital stimulation; it does not mean sex could not be physically pleasurable to them if they consented to have it. Plenty of asexual people do consider any kind of genital stimulation to be "sexual," but some asexual people make no such connection, and some understand it as a type of sexual behavior despite its being partnerless.

The same way a gay man might in some cases enjoy a sexual favor from a woman without therefore being attracted to that woman, an asexual person might enjoy a masturbatory or sexual experience—provided other factors do not repulse the person. Some asexual people enjoy the stimulation. Enjoying genital stimulation is not connected to partnered sex in everyone's mind. People of all orientations, genders, and ages may enjoy those experiences regardless of how they feel about sex.

In fact, a person doesn't even have to know what sex *is* to enjoy masturbation; three-year-olds who masturbate are unlikely to be imagining naked partners when they touch themselves, yet many young children go through a self-stimulation phase once they're out of diapers.[5] A child just knows they like how it feels. An adult will have much more context for what they're doing and will have a more complicated set of reasons for doing it, but "because it feels good" is a very simple and completely valid reason to masturbate independently of any relationship with sex.

So the presence of a sex drive, or a libido, or a desire to self-stimulate, does not disqualify someone from being asexual.[6] People do not become a certain sexual orientation based on whether they're masturbating, nor do detractors get to assign them an orientation because of misconceptions about what their behavior means. Some people who wonder whether they're asexual may think the term doesn't fit them if they desire masturbation or enjoy genital stimulation, but self-stimulation doesn't "disqualify" them.

Many asexual people describe their masturbation differently from the way other people do, though; some think of it as part of a routine to relieve stress, or they do it during a certain time of the month or day when their arousability is high, or they do it because they like the endorphins. Some may feel a building

---

5 Childhood masturbation involves stimulation of the genitals and typically begins at about two months of age, although in utero masturbatory behavior has also been reported. Incidence of this behavior typically peaks at four years of age and again in adolescence. (Yang, Fullwood, Goldstein & Mink, 2005)

6 "[M]asturbation frequency in [asexual] males was similar to available data for sexual men." (Brotto, Knudson, Inskip, Rhodes & Erskine, 2010)

need to masturbate if they don't do it for a long time, while others do it when they feel like it but don't process it as a need that has to be satisfied. Anyone may masturbate for these reasons as well.

Many asexual people who self-stimulate don't feel that masturbation is related to sex. Some argue that masturbation by definition indicates a wish to have sex, but that's not the case for everyone. Since asexual people aren't generally inspired to masturbate by attraction to other people, the connection isn't the same. Non-asexual people who masturbate may do

> "I understand that many people think of masturbation as a 'place holder' for sex, but I also know people who enjoy having sex and also enjoy masturbating just because it is an enjoyable activity in its own right and not because they just don't have sex readily available. Some asexual people fantasize while masturbating and others think about totally non-erotic things. Some people associate masturbating as a sex-drive-related release (and as an erotic behavior even though they aren't sexually attracted to others) and others think of it more as an itch to be scratched without any particular positive or negative feelings about the act. Whether or not a person masturbates doesn't change if they are sexually attracted to others or not."
> —DALLAS BRYSON, THE ASEXUAL SEXOLOGIST

so for some of the same reasons asexual people do, but they generally also still desire partnered sex; in other words, masturbation is separate from sex, and most people who do both wouldn't stop doing one if they got "enough" of the other.

And while some asexual people report having fantasies that assist their masturbation or enjoy using visual aids, many say they imagine situations they would not be comfortable with in real life or that they aren't imagining the fantasy happening to themselves. They may fantasize about a physical sensation or a sensual act, and none of this necessarily indicates that they're sexually attracted to people.

Many asexual people do describe having a low or nonexistent sex drive, though, and many don't relate to the idea of needing release through orgasm or enjoying stimulation whatsoever. The ones who have an average or even high sex drive generally still don't find themselves aroused because of attraction to someone else. Relatedly, genital reactions and arousal experiences are very common for the general population in explicitly nonsexual situations; for example, some people are embarrassed if they get an erection during a proctologist exam or when they're nervous or for no reason at all, and they will assure you that no feeling of attraction inspired that reaction in them. It's the same for asexual people who experience arousal; they may see or feel something that inspires the arousal, but the arousal does not indicate sexual attraction.

Some will argue that an asexual person who masturbates isn't asexual because the proper term would be **self-sexual** or **autosexual**; it's up to the individual what label is most appropriate, but *autosexual* generally describes behavior (referring to a person who prefers masturbation to partnered sex), which means an autosexual person could be any orientation. Again, behavior does not determine orientation.

Intimate and Sexual Activity

"When it comes to having sex with a partner, I'm largely indifferent. I don't actively seek it out. I've done it before and wasn't all that impressed, but I wouldn't necessarily be against doing it again in the right situation."

—TOM, *ASEXUALITY ARCHIVE*

Some asexual people enjoy sexual activity. Some are indifferent or ambivalent toward sex. And some are repulsed by sex. Whether an asexual person likes sex or is willing to have sex varies quite a bit and asexual people who have sex are not less legitimately asexual.

Some asexual people who enjoy sexual activity are willing to engage in sex. And some asexual people who are indifferent or ambivalent toward sex are also willing to engage in it. Asexual people who are not repulsed by being in sexual situations often describe sex as a take-it-or-leave-it activity—one that is not necessary for intimacy. And even those who enjoy the actual act will often say their motivation for doing it is primarily or partially for the benefit of the partner(s) who may consider it necessary or compelling.[7] Satisfying a partner's desire is far from the only reason an asexual person might have sex, but in many situations, sexual activity is largely influenced by the desires of an asexual person's partner(s).

So when it comes to those asexual people who are willing to have sex, why do they bother calling themselves asexual? If they're having partnered sex, what makes them still want to describe themselves with a label that supposedly implies otherwise?

Again, orientation is not the same thing as behavior. There are asexual people who have lots of sex and asexual people who have no sex and asexual people in between, but they don't become more or less asexual through their sexual experiences any more than a heterosexual person has to start identifying as bisexual or homosexual if they have a same-sex sexual experience.

---

7 "Asexuals may be willing to engage in sexually motivated behaviors to achieve nonsexual goals without experiencing sexual desire." (Prause & Graham, 2007)

The labels we choose tend to have various reasons behind them, but asexual people aren't the only types of people who are sometimes willing to have sex without sexual attraction. Some asexual people simply enjoy giving their partners something they like or they may appreciate that it's an expression of intimacy. They may value the closeness sex brings to their relationship or they may be curious about the experience and aren't so put off by it that they're unwilling to try. They may also enjoy the physical act itself in a sensual way, or they may want to have sex for procreation. Plenty of people who aren't asexual might relate to having sex for these reasons too.

All that said, it's much more common for an asexual person to be totally unwilling or reluctant to have sex. Relationships can still succeed even if a person can't or won't have sex; after all, plenty of people who aren't asexual have reasons they can't or won't have sex (disability or health conditions that prevent it, for instance). Though it is sometimes a hurdle, there is no hard and fast rule that relationships must include sex to become long term or to sustain sufficient intimacy.

For the majority of repulsed or reluctant asexual people, it's only the idea or experience of *personally* being in a sexual situation that seems unappealing; some of this group will be sickened by images of sex like pornography, love scenes, or explicit public displays of affection, but nearly all are supportive of others' wish to have sex as long as they themselves do not have to be involved. In other words, being a repulsed asexual person is not defined as thinking sex is a disgusting concept in general, and it's not about thinking sex is evil, wrong, or destructive. (This response exists too, but it is not definitive of sex-repulsed asexuality.)

In a survey of 3,436 self-identified asexual-spectrum people administered on the Internet in September–October 2011, respondents offered the following attitudes toward the idea or experience of having sex:[8]	
I am **completely repulsed** by the idea of (myself) having sex	17.0%
I am **somewhat repulsed** by the idea of (myself) having sex	40.1%
I am **indifferent** to the idea of (myself) having sex	35.7%
I **would not be willing** to have sex	26.0%
I **would be willing** to compromise and have **occasional** sex (in a relationship)	35.9%
I **would be willing** to compromise and have **regular** sex (in a relationship)	17.0%
I **enjoy** having sex	6.9%

* Participants were allowed to choose more than one answer.

8 Community Census. (Asexual Awareness Week, 2011)

So why won't a self-described repulsed asexual person be "open-minded" enough to just try sex?

Many non-asexual people aren't willing to try sex with someone they're not at all attracted to, and this is usually considered reasonable. And yet, suddenly when it's asexual people in question, they are often considered unreasonable for saying no for the same reason. Asexual people shouldn't be expected to experiment with sex "just to make sure," because asexuality only means they are not sexually attracted to others. Calling oneself asexual does *not* mean they know without trying that it's impossible for them to enjoy a sex act, but enjoying a sex act would not make them stop being asexual.

Imagine the case of a heterosexual man who is not attracted to other men in the least. He can know he has no attraction to men without trying to have sex with them because his feelings of disinterest or repulsion are very likely to prevent him from enjoying the experience. He does not feel he needs to have sex with a man to prove he is not attracted to men or to be sure that he wouldn't enjoy it. He is trusted, without trying it, to understand, express, and live according to his own feelings. And he is not accused of being close-minded due to unwillingness to try sex with a man, nor is he frequently told by mainstream voices what great gay sex he is missing.

Repulsed asexual people should be similarly respected. It's not helpful to teach them they should be indifferent enough to ignore their own feelings. **Asexual people aren't a special category of people who will benefit from being badgered into trying sex against their inclinations.** Some people are repulsed at the idea of having sex with someone who isn't attractive to them, and when a person is asexual, no one is sexually attractive. It's just the way they are.

Moving away from specifically sexual activity: what about cuddling, spooning, kissing, or sensual touch? As previously stated, asexual people are as varied as the rest of the population in their answers to whether they will accept and enjoy these experiences. Many people

"I like touching people. Platonically, mostly. I like holding hands, and I like hugging, and I like cuddling, and I like sitting back-to-back, and I like sitting next to people so that our knees touch, and lots and lots of other things. I call the inclination to touch people 'sensual attraction' even though there are bunches of other senses, because 'physical attraction' tends to make people think of lust. And it is a lust! Just not a sex-related one, which is the connotation most people have with lust when not given context."

—ANONYMOUS, ASEXUAL TUMBLR USER

who may not enjoy or desire sex still like physical closeness; they may experience **sensual attraction** to others and enjoy touching, but that experience does not inspire sexual attraction. (For non-asexual people, sensual enjoyment and sensual attraction can of course be experienced in addition to sexual attraction, but it can happen independently of it too, just like romantic attraction can.)

People who like intimate closeness may like to snuggle, hug, lie together, or give/get massages or other kinds of nonsexual touch, and some asexual people enjoy those activities. Also, what constitutes "sexual" is not always the same from partnership to partnership. There are plenty of asexual people who enjoy kissing and feel satisfied with the sensual aspect of it but don't experience a sexual attraction toward the partner they're kissing. It can be confusing and frustrating when partners who have different needs may believe "one thing leads to another," but it's just not true in all cases. It should be noted that an asexual person is not being a tease through the act of enjoying kissing or sensual touch but not wanting to include sex.

Polyamory and Non-Monogamy

Sometimes asexual people are comfortable as members of polyamorous groups and other non-monogamies. There are many reasons why an asexual person might find a non-monogamous relationship more comfortable than having a single monogamous partner:

- They may have varied emotional or practical needs that are better satisfied by more than one person
- They may prefer to eschew traditional arrangements of commitment
- They may feel more secure knowing that their non-asexual partner(s) can get sexual satisfaction without needing it from them (thus sparing them possible guilt and sparing any non-asexual partners possible frustration)

These situations are not without challenges, though; communication can clear up most misconceptions, but some polyamorous or non-monogamous asexual people may find themselves less included or regarded as outsiders if they don't participate in sex, sexual activities, or sexual discussions; they may also face misconceptions from outside if they or their partner(s) are interpreted as "cheating." Negotiating non-monogamies can be difficult in a culture that expects relationships to be primarily built around sex and exclusive pair-bonding, but sometimes opening a relationship to include additional people or allowing partners to pursue connections outside the relationship can solve problems for the right people.

Kink, Fetish Play, and BDSM

Can asexual people have kinks? Enjoy fetish play? Engage in BDSM (Bondage/Discipline, Dominance/submission, Sadism/masochism)? Yes, they can. These practices and proclivities are often explicitly associated with sex, but they can still be enjoyed by asexual people in ways that do not require sexual attraction or sexual activity. Sometimes a focus on sex—perceived or actual—in BDSM spaces discourages some kinky asexual people from exploring or continuing to engage, but there are also plenty of opportunities that are safe and satisfying for asexual people, even if they're sex-repulsed.

In fact, many non-asexual people who engage in BDSM derive at least some of their pleasure from experiences that don't depend on sexual attraction to any partner(s). Asexual people can enjoy kinky experiences or have fetishes independently of attraction, and in some cases independently of sexual arousal or interest, though what constitutes "sexual" in these contexts is sometimes not as clear-cut as one might expect.

For instance, in Dominance/submission, the thrill of Dominance or being submissive doesn't necessarily depend on any genital contact, and it is not necessarily a sexual experience or sexual reward. So much of BDSM and fetish play depends on the psychological stimulation participants enjoy through consensual roleplay acts; sex or sexual attraction doesn't necessarily even have to be a part of the experience to be satisfying. When an object or body part or roleplay experience is focused upon in a fetish situation, sometimes sexual attraction to the partner(s) is absent or unnecessary—and sometimes these experiences can be partnerless.

Even people who are not asexual can sometimes prefer or enjoy BDSM that is carried out with a partner they are not sexually attracted to, and it's relatively common for a session to be carried out completely focused on an experience other than sex, especially in the case of some professional BDSM practitioners who choose not to have sex with clients. Giving or receiving pain, bondage, or service in these consensual situations is sometimes described as an endorphin rush that kinky folks enjoy on a level that can be comparable to sex, and some rewards are delivered verbally through interactive scenes, consensually invoked verbal punishment, or spoken praise/positive reinforcement.

In some relationships that involve kink, far more than just a couple of partners are involved. Sometimes groups are formed around an activity or group of activities that all the members enjoy, carry out, and play together, and this is enjoyable even between members of the group who are not sexually attracted to or involved with each other. An asexual kinkster might participate in this sort of atmosphere and be quite satisfied. Despite what some people think, BDSM and kink communities are famously respectful of consensual and respectful interaction (even if the practices and scenes themselves might involve punishment and pain). If an asexual person wants a kinky experience without sexual contact, they will usually be able to find something satisfying for them.

Asexual people with kinks and fetishes are a minority, but acknowledging them is important, and their interests don't invalidate other aspects of their identities. One of the most well-known fetish communities online—fetlife.com—has some sections devoted to asexual folks ("Asexual & Kinky"[9]; "Ace BDSM Support Group"[10]), and an asexuality-specific fetish organization exists.[11]

Gray Areas

For some people, sexual identity is very simple. It fits easily into well-defined boxes and is uncomplicated to describe. It's not confusing to experience because it's common and well represented in culture and media; it's easy to know what to look for in a partner; the sorts of sexual experiences the relationship might lead to are predictable.

But gray areas exist in all orientations. Let's use heterosexuality for an example: say there's a person who identifies as heterosexual. This person spends most of their life only attracted to cross-gender partners . . . but once or twice has feelings for a member of the same gender. Depending on that person's related feelings about homosexuality and availability of potential partners, they may or may not experiment. Are they therefore considered bisexual from then on?

No, a person in this situation does not have to identify as bisexual—not unless they think that's an important label to use. If those people find it useful to say "I lean hetero, but am technically bi," great. If they find that "straight" fits their attraction experiences more accurately, they should be able to identify as straight without argument. Sexual orientation is a continuum, and the labels people choose are useful only to the extent that they communicate what we want them to.

Graysexuality

So, just like with our heterosexual person who has had one or two same-sex attractions, it stands to reason that some people fall very close to asexual but occasionally do experience sexual attraction. Some might say those people are "just picky." Some might say they "just have low sex drive" (even though some people on the asexual spectrum have average or high sex drives). But feeling

---

9 Asexual & Kinky on *FetLife*: fetlife.com/groups/7247
10 Ace BDSM Support Group on *FetLife*: fetlife.com/groups/41247
11 *Ace Fet*: www.acefet.org/

attracted to others isn't something a person chooses, and many people in this middle-ground situation have a lot more in common with asexual people than with non-asexual people because they expect their relationships to not involve sexual attraction, don't see their relationships in terms of sexual attraction, or very rarely experience sexual attraction.

Some people who have this in-between experience call themselves **graysexual, gray-asexual, gray-A, gray ace,** or **grace**, short for the gray area of sexuality. It's a useful term for those who primarily live with an asexual experience of the world, but can experience or have experienced sexual attraction and wish to acknowledge it in their label. This is not

> "Because I am gray-A, I am between orientations. That does not necessarily mean that I am fluidly switching back and forth between allosexual and asexual. It's not like I'm asexual for most of the year, but the local ace meetup group has to avoid scheduling on full moons. No, I feel sort-of-not-really-attracted to people on a daily basis."
>
> —Tristan Miller, *The Asexual Agenda*

the same as "grayromantic"; this refers to one's *sexual* orientation, not one's romantic orientation.

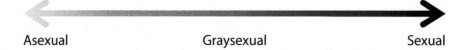

Asexual   Graysexual   Sexual

Just like with grayromanticism, graysexuality can be combined with another orientation descriptor. Some examples:

A graysexual heteroromantic person: Is rarely/occasionally sexually attracted to others and experiences cross-gender romantic attraction more typically.

An asexual grayromantic person: Is not sexually attracted to anyone but has an occasional/rare experience of being romantically attracted to others.

A graysexual homoromantic person: Is rarely/occasionally sexually attracted to others and is romantically attracted to others of the same gender.

A gray-pansexual aromantic person: Is rarely/occasionally sexually attracted to people of all genders but is never romantically attracted to anyone.

A gynesexual gray-biromantic person: Is sexually attracted to women and/or feminine-presenting people, and occasionally/rarely experiences romantic attraction toward more than one gender.

It can seem a little confusing with all the mix-and-match, but most people who use very specific terms like this are trying to talk about their attraction experiences in detail and figure out/discuss a pattern. People may use these words in academic or advanced-level sexuality contexts, but in casual conversation it's more likely that a pansexual gray-homoromantic woman's description of herself will sound more like "I think all genders are sexy, but I only seem to fall in love with other women, and it's rare." Most people in asexual communities don't feel the need to be this specific about the "rules" of their attraction experiences, but the words are there for the people who want to have detailed discussions.

Graysexuality is an umbrella term. It can refer to many situations wherein a person is experiencing something that isn't as consistent, as strong, as predictable, or as prevalent as most other people experience it. Graysexual folks won't all describe their feelings the same way. Here are some descriptions graysexual people might use:

- They feel sexual attraction, but it's weak
- They go through phases of feeling sexual attraction and phases of not feeling it
- They feel attractions but are unsure of whether they are sexual attractions
- They get caught up in a partner's sexual desire and enjoy it vicariously but don't feel it intrinsically
- They find only a tiny sliver of the population sexually attractive
- They find people sexy but have no physical reaction to them
- They find people sexy but are unable or unwilling to pursue someone as a partner

All of these are not-exactly-asexual ways of viewing other people, but are outside the widely accepted norms of non-asexual people.

Not everyone who is somewhere in the gray area feels like it needs a term; they may be fine with calling themselves picky or saying their sexual attraction is too weak for them to care much or that the kind of people they're attracted to aren't plentiful. But some may feel comfortable using the label as a way to explain the difference between what they're feeling and how most others describe their attraction experience.

An anonymous gray-asexual panromantic person's perspective on the gray areas:

"Imagine full sexuality as a glass of soda and asexuality as a glass of water. To the person with the water, it tastes like plain water, and they're happy with that as long as soda-drinkers don't insist they should like soda. Likewise, the people with various flavors of soda will be happy with them and be able to identify them as soda, even though some of them might be 'mixed flavors' of varying percentages that are hard to pick out. Some may even have some ice melted in them, but as long as it's not much, well, it's still a soda. But my case is like having a glass of water with a little bit of soda poured into it. When I taste it, I can't really tell what's off about it. It doesn't seem like just water, but it's definitely not a cup of soda. I might not even be able to identify the off taste as soda. Maybe it's not! Sometimes I think I taste it more than others. But I'm not sure I like the taste of it. It's confusing, and it might be easier if I just had a glass of plain water, but I don't really have any control over that. But overall, I still feel like what I have is much more like water than soda, especially since I can't always even identify the added ingredient as soda. So I'll call it water. Just not plain water."

Demisexuality

We all know it's possible for some people to be immediately sexually attracted to other people based on information gathered with one's physical senses—without knowing anything about their personalities. It can be based on looks or voice or chemistry or charisma, and it's known as a **primary sexual attraction** reaction. That person seems like a good sex partner, and there's a physical and/or mental sexual reaction. It doesn't mean one is necessarily *realistically* interested in sex with that person or is ready to run into the nearest closet for a quickie. It just means there is a reaction that is sexual—that a person can be seen in a sexual context even as a stranger.

Secondary sexual attraction is more gradual, though not inherently a "different kind" of sexual attraction—it just happens under different circumstances. A partner starts to seem sexually appealing only after an emotional bond develops (not necessarily love), based on qualities that can't be perceived through immediate observation of the subject without interaction. This can happen in conjunction with primary sexual attraction, combining with it, enhancing it. But some people *only* experience that slow, less reactionary rise of interest—they never experience primary or immediate sexual attraction and can't feel attraction to strangers or celebrities they don't know. Some people who only experience sexual attraction after developing a bond with someone find it useful to call themselves **demisexual**.

As with graysexuality and grayromanticism, demisexual is not the same thing as demiromantic; demisexual people are experiencing *sexual* attraction under these circumstances, and demiromantic folks are experiencing *romantic* attraction. A person can be both demisexual and demiromantic, but every combination exists: heterosexual/demiromantic; demisexual/aromantic; homosexual/demi-biromantic—the list goes on. Any mixture of sexual orientation and romantic orientation can exist, though asexual communities are probably the places you'll see it the most because they tend to be one of the major groups that almost always needs to separate their sexual orientation from their romantic orientation to make sense of it.

The notion of primary versus secondary sexual attraction is hotly debated by some people who think acknowledging demisexuality is a way of shaming people who experience and express their sexuality more normatively. Most of the time this is based on a misconception that secondary sexual attraction is being billed as "meaningful" or "authentic" while primary sexual attraction is "animalistic" or "shallow." However, in reality, neither type is being defined as more valuable or meaningful or more "real"; most people experience both types, meaning they might have an initial (primary) sexual attraction to a person but develop an additional (secondary) type of sexual attraction because of who that person is—developing from familiarity, specific turn-ons, past memories, et cetera.

Some also think that *demisexuality* isn't a meaningful term because some people—especially women—are rewarded with social approval for having sex only after the emotional bond develops. Since they're supposedly expected to do this, some critics say demisexual people must think *most* sexual relationships aren't meaningful or don't require emotion, while their own are and do.

But demisexuality isn't about willingness to have sex. It's about capacity to experience sexual attraction. Some demisexual people *do* have sex without the emotional connection just like anyone in the larger population might. **A demisexual label doesn't describe whether a person has sex, nor does it suggest a person embraces any particular ideology regarding sex.** It just means the person sometimes has the capacity to develop sexual attraction if and only if other bonds develop first. Whether these folks have sex is a choice, but whether they experience sexual attraction is not a choice. Their orientation is not about sex moralism.

In a survey of 3,436 self-identified asexual-spectrum people administered on the Internet in September–October 2011, respondents offered the following answers when asked "How do you identify on the asexual spectrum?"[12]

Asexual	65.2%
Demisexual	20.6%
Gray-asexual	26.3%
Other	5.3%

* Participants were allowed to choose more than one answer.

When demisexual people only experience sexual attraction to those with whom they've developed a bond, they may be experiencing the world in a primarily asexual way, so they are usually considered to be on the asexual spectrum. But demisexual people often hear others say there's nothing asexual about demisexuality because their experience is actually the way sexual attraction works for the majority.

> "Your friends will only accept so many 'I like him as a friend's before you give up and claim to 'like like' someone at random. As if that weren't awkward enough, you then have to justify your 'like like' in what amounts to a foreign language—'I really like . . . his . . . nose? No? No, of course I don't like his nose. I like his . . . Star Wars t-shirt? No, obviously not. His . . . book report about Huck Finn?'"
> —REBECCA

Those on the asexual spectrum tend to disagree. They see their peers finding movie stars and cute strangers hot and don't relate to it at all, because they don't experience it. Getting excited over a sexy celebrity may seem nonsensical and baffling to a demisexual person, and those who acknowledge that sexual attraction to strangers is very common can't turn around and say "most people aren't ever attracted to strangers." Some detractors don't understand why "I'm attracted to others, but only with an emotional connection" needs its own sexual orientation.

To understand demisexuality, one just needs to realize that demisexual people aren't identifying that way to shame anyone or separate themselves from a "lower" form of sexual interest. They're describing how sexual attraction works for them, and observing that it's different from the way it works for most because they have no concept of "do you think that person's hot?" just based on how someone looks, sounds, smells, or moves. (Many asexual

---

12 Community Census. (Asexual Awareness Week, 2011)

people have this bewildering experience in adolescence—being asked by friends to state whether someone is attractive and having no idea what they're supposed to feel, perhaps hiding their confusion by pretending to be attracted to whoever everyone else calls hot. Demisexual people experience this too.)

It's also inaccurate to say demisexual people are claiming not to be aroused by the physical. They certainly can be. They can feel sexually attracted to the physical attributes of a person they have an emotional connection with, but they will never feel sexual attraction to a stranger even if they have those same physical attributes. The distinction is sometimes difficult for others to grasp, but demisexual people feel it is there, and they aren't doing it to put their sexual attraction experience on a pedestal. Whether to call oneself "demisexual" is ultimately up to the person in question, dependent upon whether it is useful.

Asexual Relationships

As mentioned previously, some asexual people want committed relationships.

Most people assume that if an asexual person wants a relationship, the course of action that makes the most sense is to find another asexual person and have a sexless relationship. However, finding an asexual partner isn't as simple a solution as it sounds.

First of all, asexuality is relatively uncommon, and as of this writing, so is awareness about it. Most asexual folks don't know using the asexual label is an option for much of their lives, which limits their ability to find others. Even if they choose to come out and discuss it publicly, they are often the only asexual person in their social group. Asexual people can meet each other serendipitously in ordinary social interactions, but more often, if they want to meet others, they have to do it deliberately. Possible partners can be found on the Internet, but the issues involved in relationships that are likely to be long distance tend to make a happy outcome less likely to occur. Asexual people are just not anywhere near as likely to run into each other, and there's no Asexual Night at the club.

So asexual people have a small and scattered asexual partner pool to begin with, and then on top of that they have all the same compatibility issues that anyone else looking for a relationship has. Asexual folks want to find partners who complement them, and finding partners with the right traits and common interests is sometimes more important to them than compatibility in the bedroom. Sexual compatibility is not always the first thing on a person's mind in partner searches. An asexual/asexual relationship is not automatically an ideal situation just because they're more likely to be compatible sexually, any more than any two same-gender people are perfect for each other if they're both gay. In short, it just isn't practical for all partner-seeking asexual people to specify that their partners must also be asexual.

In addition, not all relationships become romantic partnerships deliberately; sometimes asexual people and non-asexual people fall in love or partner up even though they weren't looking to do so (possibly before the asexual people know they're asexual), and while they obviously weren't *trying* to create a complicated situation, they now have to figure out how they're going to handle it.

Obviously—like any relationship—these relationships require compromise. Sometimes people of any orientation will make compromises that are unrelated to sex, such as deciding to move to a new place to be close to a long-distance significant other or putting up with other incompatibilities because they value a different aspect of the relationship more. But with asexual people, the question of how they'll handle sex and intimacy in relationships is often at the forefront of everyone's mind.

If the sexual needs in a relationship are mismatched, many will assign the blame for the mismatch to the asexual partner(s) in any relationship.[13] Some see this couple or this group as problematic because "the asexual person doesn't want sex enough," not because "the sexual needs here are mismatched." To begin to understand these compatibility issues, it must first be acknowledged that **every arrangement is different and the ultimate purpose should never be "how can we change the asexual person?"**

Some people protest that non-asexual people should not have to share any of the responsibility for the incompatibility because sex is expected in a normal relationship. It is owed to them; it is understood to be part of the package deal. If someone feels they cannot be in a relationship in which their partner(s) might not consider sex a must, they should not date an asexual person who's reluctant toward or repulsed by sex. Asexual people are regularly subjected to expectations for sex they may not want to fulfill, and sometimes their possible insecurity over this sensitive issue is exploited.

Asexual people in relationships—especially women—face coercion and are at higher risk for sexual assault, which is often overlooked because outside observers may believe the aggressor deserves sex or that people who are in relationships are in a constant state of consent and therefore are not capable of sexually assaulting each other. Anyone who has relationships with asexual people should try to be particularly aware of the way societal expectations may translate to

---

13 "Someone who is incapable of meeting a sexual's needs has no business dating a sexual in the first place, if you ask me. At the very least, asexuality must be disclosed." Dan Savage on relationships involving asexual people. (Savage, 2009)

internal relationship expectations in ways that can damage and abuse any partner who doesn't desire sex or isn't willing to engage in it.

Be aware that there is nothing wrong with considering sex necessary in your relationship. That's fine—**it's your right to specify what the boundaries and dealbreakers of your relationship are and what expressions of intimacy you're looking for**. But relationship-seeking people should try to express their desires as "their preferences," not as "the way things are supposed to be" (therefore attempting to justify demands that only asexual partners be required to compromise).

If an asexual person wants a relationship with someone who *does* want to make sex part of the relationship, compromise is in order. Here are some ways that couples or groups with different sexual needs involving at least one asexual person have handled their relationships.

1. Sometimes a partner with sexual needs is willing to give up sex for an asexual partner and either ignores sexual urges or takes care of sexual urges through masturbation.
2. Sometimes the partners agree to have occasional or regular sex, depending on the degree of tolerance for or interest in sex the asexual person has.
3. Sometimes the partners agree to an open relationship or open marriage in which partners who want to can have other partners.
4. Sometimes an asexual person is part of a polyamorous group in which the other partners have their sexual needs satisfied with each other.[14]
5. Sometimes the partner(s) with sexual needs can be satisfied by physically intimate play that does not cross any intimacy lines set down by any partner(s); some asexual people enjoy or allow kissing, cuddling, making out, petting, kink/BDSM/fetish play, or stimulating a partner manually or using toys.

If a compromise can't be reached or someone is unhappy with the compromises after trying them out, it's okay to acknowledge that some partnerships can't work. Breakups can of course involve frustration and bitterness, and sometimes the ex-partners will carry guilt regarding their inability to make their partner(s) happy, but any partnership needs to take an honest look at the partners' needs and recognize if they are ill-equipped to meet them. The decision to go your separate ways for each of your own good can be a self-affirming and healthy

---

14 "[S]ome asexual identified individuals describe current or idealized relationships that fit definitions of polyamorous relationships." (Scherrer K. S., 2009)

experience and shouldn't necessarily be seen as a failure or "proof" that these types of relationships never work.

Even if partners must end a relationship that turns out to be incompatible, they can still treasure the time they had together and consider it a growing experience. Every relationship will involve big issues to work out—sex is only one of them—and partnerships might just as likely involve compromise or breakups if the partners had different opinions on having children or sharing their living space.

Asexual people do often feel guilty if they don't satisfy their partners in a way that seems so fundamental and important to them. This happens even without inordinate pressure from the partners or society. No one likes to be a disappointment, and asexual people are (sadly) pretty used to being treated like they are not good enough for a partner because of this "flaw." They may be tempted to stay in less-than-healthy relationships because they believe they will never find anyone else who will tolerate their peculiarities or because they know how rare it is to find potential partners who share or respect their desires (or lack thereof).

Those who do feel sexual attraction or interest and find themselves in a relationship (or potential relationship) with asexual people should try to understand that their asexual partners aren't trying to make them unhappy. If there's something the asexual partners can give that they're willing to do and it does not violate terms any partner holds dear, it can still be a satisfying relationship. Communication is key, and non-asexual people should attempt to understand that asexual people are frequently led to believe they are undesirable and unworthy of love. They may need some extra reassurance if their asexuality or level of sexual willingness is not a dealbreaker; they may secretly fear their non-asexual partners will eventually leave them over this.

Considering it's common in relationships to have different sexual appetites, quirks, desires, kinks, and preferences, all relationships contain this element of compromise to some degree. **A relationship with an asexual person is not necessarily all or nothing**. More help for asexual people on relationships with non-asexual people can be found in Part Four of this book. Help for non-asexual people who want to be good partners to asexual people and find happiness themselves can be found in Part Five.

Some asexual people do get married or have long-term relationships. It's not impossible, and it's not ridiculous. They may or may not want children. They may or may not want a monogamous relationship. They may or may not want their relationships to involve emotional attraction. They may or may not like physical intimacy, and they should be trusted to navigate these avenues themselves even though it can be difficult.

Sometimes asexual people get married and tolerate sex they may not desire because they've been taught they're supposed to want it, believing it's just part of being a good spouse. There have been incidents in asexual communities of married asexual people finding out about asexuality and realizing "Hey, lots of people have felt the way I feel," and it may lead them to negotiate their relationship differently. Unfortunately this does sometimes lead to marital strife and subsequent breakups, but this is generally only in the case of people who insist their (newly discovered) asexual partner must continue to have sex against their will or as part of a perceived "duty" in the marriage.

If a previously happy marriage dissolves over this, of course it's sad, but an asexual person who feels newly empowered to refuse unwanted sex shouldn't be attacked for "ruining the relationship." After all, if an asexual person was having regular sex because they felt they were obligated to and that they had no power to refuse, this relationship was dependent upon exploiting a lopsided power dynamic, and that calls into question whether the consent was valid and whether the relationship was appropriate in the first place. If a critic argues that the relationship was "happy" *when the asexual person felt required to hide and be ashamed of their lack of desire*, that critic is suggesting that only one person—the non-asexual person—actually has desires that matter in the relationship.

Chances are the asexual person will still want other needs met and will desire other forms of intimacy, and some of those may be physical; the partners should discuss how they'd like to move forward, this time with an asexual partner's boundaries and desires given just as much priority as a non-asexual partner's.

Sometimes relationship therapy does help. However, partnered people should be aware that not all sex therapists or relationship therapists recognize asexuality as an orientation, and it's possible they may approach less willing partners as the only "problem children." If someone's relationship therapy focuses entirely on how to help an asexual person tolerate or initiate sex more often to satisfy someone with a larger sexual appetite, it is not balanced therapy. Pushing someone into unwanted sex and telling them they should like it is abuse. Unless the asexual person has expressed a wish to cultivate an interest in or a tolerance for sexual activity, this is not appropriate and they should find another therapist.

Society, Discrimination, and Queer Communities

Some asexual people feel comfortable allying with or joining communities dedicated to supporting people of marginalized sexualities, romantic orientations, and genders.

Many LGBTQ communities open their arms to any non-heteronormative[15] individual or group in need of a place to belong. **Some asexual-spectrum people and their allies feel asexuality is inherently queer, while some believe the term is inaccurate or don't personally identify with it**.

Asexual people allying with queer communities are learning about inclusivity, fellowship, organization of marginalized groups, and visibility, and they are also offering valuable insights to queer organizations, regardless of whether any individual thinks asexual people should be recognized as members.

Because of asexual people's rarity, it's not always practical for them to expect thriving local communities just based on asexuality, though meetup groups have worked in some places. As of this writing, there aren't whole physical organizations dedicated to asexual support; there's no Asexual Night at local clubs; there are no Asexual Studies courses at colleges (though once in a while it gets touched on in a curriculum[16]). This is part of the reason why some asexual people feel comfortable joining or working with local LGBTQ chapters or Gay/Straight Alliances (GSAs); people who are non-normative in sexuality, romantic orientation, or gender tend to have some of the same problems and experiences asexual people do and might be able to understand other forms of discrimination and alienation more readily.

However, it should be noted that **even though non-asexual-spectrum queer individuals can be marginalized because of their sexual orientation, they do share with heterosexual people the experience of sexual attraction and may not necessarily understand why asexual people would belong (or want to belong) in their spaces**. As mentioned, many *do* support asexuality, just like many asexual people are allies of LGBTQ folks and support their rights. But some members of these groups do argue that asexuality is not inherently queer and that the only asexual people who would belong in an LGBTQ group are LGBT asexual people. Heteroromantic and aromantic cisgender asexual people are sometimes unwelcome.[17]

There are two sides to this story, and each organization and each person will have to come to an individual conclusion.

On asexual people having a space in queer groups, regardless of whether asexuality is inherently queer:

---

15 *Heteronormative* refers to norms about a person's lifestyle that dictate acceptance and assumption of heterosexuality, cisgender identity, and traditional gender roles.

16 The Asexual Sexologist offers asexuality-related materials for use in sexuality courses. (Asexual Sexologist, 2012)

17 Allison Hope examined whether asexuality is queer in her *Huffington Post* article "Does Asexuality Fall Under the Queer Umbrella?" The comments sometimes agreed that asexual people belong, and sometimes insisted that asexual people experience no discrimination and therefore do not deserve support from LGBT organizations. (Hope, 2012)

Asexual people are not the same as heterosexual people who aren't having sex, which is what some misunderstand them as. There is a difference between an abstinent heterosexual person and an asexual person: abstinence is a practice (a choice), while asexuality is an orientation (not a choice—a familiar distinction for LGBTQ folks). Asexual people don't face the same oppression (unless they are asexual *and* some form of LGBT), but even heteroromantic asexual people are not having "the heterosexual experience" either. Just like many LGBTQ people, asexual people still have to deal with fighting society's expectations and developing pride and confidence in their orientation.

Active persecution of asexual people is usually fairly invisible to the outside observer—with the exception of specific educational efforts that attract uninformed, superficial hatred and an influx of dismissive, invalidating strangers purporting to be motivated by "concern" for asexual people's happiness. [Author's note: large-scale attacks have happened to me at least a dozen times as an asexual activist, though only two of the stalking/harassing attempts were serious enough that I had to pursue legal action.] And as with most articles featuring LGBTQ topics, one only needs to read the comments section on an asexuality article to see the overwhelming ignorance and hatred people are willing to spew on the subject of asexual people and their perceived "brokenness."

By and large, the message asexual people get from society is that they do not exist and/or that they should get help to change themselves; if they do not try every possible avenue to become another sexual orientation, they deserve what they get. When the overarching master narrative of society dictates that "being fully human" or "being a complete person" is dependent on experiencing sexual attraction, there are specialized situations in which asexual people can be actively persecuted/disliked *for* being asexual,[18] and that is rarely taken into account by those who want to exclude them from queer spaces.

Though asexual people are treated similarly to LGBTQ people in certain situations if their orientation is known, for most asexual folks **it's not an experience of outward oppression so much as it's an experience of omission—of being left out and unable to participate in something that's supposedly central to life**.

Some say an asexual person would have to disclose their orientation to receive any kind of negative reaction, but that isn't true since the heteronormative

---

18 "Attitudes toward homosexuals, bisexuals, and asexuals were more negative than attitudes toward heterosexuals, revealing a sexual minority bias. Within sexual minorities, homosexuals were evaluated most positively, followed by bisexuals, with asexuals being evaluated most negatively of all groups. [. . .] A sexual minority bias was evident, whereby participants were most willing to rent to and/ or hire heterosexuals relative to homosexuals, bisexuals, or asexuals." (MacInnis & Hodson, 2012)

assumption encourages most people to perceive them as non-participating, flawed, or repressed heterosexual people. Aromantic asexual people go through life with people of all orientations making certain assumptions about their failure to find romantic partners, and romantic asexual people are repeatedly sent messages about how dysfunctional their relationships must be if sex isn't involved or desired. The damaging messages might even come from asexual people's partner(s), and they tend to have far worse effects than most outside the experience imagine—especially if those affected do not have resources and support.

Some will say that enduring invisibility isn't the same as "oppression"—and they're right, though what *happens* as a result of systematic erasure, verbal abuse, and misunderstanding can be oppressive. LGBTQ people do experience oppression in the forms of fearing and/or experiencing hate crimes, being denied certain rights that are afforded to cisgender heterosexual people, being discriminated against, and being openly mocked. Asexual people are less likely to experience these specific forms of oppression on the basis of their orientation—except for mocking, and the mocking sounds different—though in certain situations asexual people can be uniquely discriminated against. (This will be discussed shortly.)

Asexual people aren't saying they have an identical or worse experience when compared to LGBTQ people. Asexual people are saying they often feel omitted, erased, and excluded and that they move through life facing consistent challenges to their sexual orientation.

"The first time I saw the bit about asexuals passing for straight so easily, I was a bit flabbergasted. Because I don't pass as straight for any length of time. My experience throughout high school always came back to carefully guarded questions and tentative attempts to get me to come out. And those were the polite ones."

—Sciatrix, *Writing From Factor X*

Asexual people usually don't appreciate being told their experience is analogous to a heterosexual person's experience. Non-asexual people don't know what it's like to be asexual. They may not know what it's like to be honest about one's orientation only to be told such a thing isn't real, isn't happening, isn't possible. While well-known physical organizations dedicated to supporting LGBTQ communities exist, with loads of resources and information, asexual people usually aren't included in the outreach or represented in the queer library materials. Asexual people have fewer places to turn for information or community or support, and the absence of organizations to foster their health and happiness helps contribute to the message that they do not exist. It is an insidious form of exclusion and it can be damaging.

LGBTQ people are regularly subjected to cruel messages, of course—which can result in a person defaulting to self-hate or self-doubt because of the abundant messages from outside—so they may share plenty of common ground with asexual people. They can all have coming-out experiences and sometimes receive misguided messages that they need therapy, haven't met the right partner, or are going against/failing to fulfill an obligation in their religion.

So, it's important to remember that "not-LGB" does not equal "heterosexual." Asexual people are subjected to many assumptions about their sexuality that can easily wear down their self-esteem and force them to question whether they can trust their own feelings, and—this is key—they are much rarer than LGB people, so it is vital that every effort be made to respect asexual people's desire to access community.

It is damaging and erasing to tell asexual people that being assumed heterosexual and experiencing heterosexual privilege *is really the same as being heterosexual* (and therefore they shouldn't expect and shouldn't get help or understanding and are stepping on toes by hoping to access support). This is especially true considering there are plenty of gay folks who aren't readily recognized as gay (but they're not less deserving of support) and plenty of trans folks who are not read as trans (but don't stop needing community support if they are usually mistaken for cisgender).

Having most people assume you're heterosexual means being treated like you're heterosexual when you're not, and while being treated heterosexual and "normal" does bring certain privileges, it is also alienating and erasing when it doesn't fit one's comfort level and participation with heterosexual culture and identity.

If an asexual person is saying "I'm queer," they may be using the broad definition of queer, meaning "I'm not heteronormative in my sexual orientation and/or gender." If an LGBTQ person has a stricter definition of what *queer* means, they may be hesitant to open

> "I find it painfully ironic that in queer spaces I am still told that my sexual orientation is just a disorder, either physical or psychological, that I 'just haven't met the right person yet,' that I'm going through a phase, that I can be cured. I hardly consider a space where people feel comfortable saying those things to another person a 'safe space' for anyone (and yes, they say those things to me as a polypan ace (. . .) and those same things are said to trans* aces and homoromantic aces and biromantic aces, too)."
> —DALLAS BRYSON, *THE ASEXUAL SEXOLOGIST*

the arms of their queer community to a person who isn't LGBT, but if they attempt to understand each asexual person's reason for identifying as queer, they may conclude that some or all of them belong under the umbrella.

Some may say asexual people don't have problems (or the right problems, or enough problems), and therefore they should just go ally with heterosexual people, but this ignores the fact that heteronormative attitudes influence the heterosexual world to also exclude asexual people. If "not LGB" is understood to mean "heterosexual" in queer spaces, those who say so are processing heterosexual as the default, which is an attitude that also hurts them. Even aromantic asexual people, who are less likely to be assumed heterosexual because they are unlikely to have romantic partners, are sometimes told "you don't belong here because you're just straight." Perceived blank spaces being interpreted as heterosexual by default is a heteronormative assumption.

If any asexual person who participates in an LGBTQ community or one of its organizations ends up behaving problematically, that can be addressed on an individual level—just like it would be if any other person was dominating the discussion or making others feel unsafe. All queer communities have the capacity to have problematic members, and some individuals with more relative privilege may make the space feel unsafe for other individuals even if they "qualify" with a letter in the acronym. Evaluating on a case-by-case basis often works better than denying access to all heteroromantic or aromantic asexual people as a rule (especially if the queer group in question accepts allies in its meetings and membership).

"The real question is, are there spaces that asexuals and LGBT people can share? Should there be? Does this particular configuration help people? Language has an effect on this question. If asexuals think of themselves as just allies, they will be less likely to participate or share their own experiences. Is that what we want? If an asexual acts homophobic, or an LGBT person hates on aces, do we want to treat it as an attack from the outside, or as ignorance from the inside?"
—Tristan Miller, Skeptic's Play

After all, not all LGBTQ people are equally oppressed; one must take into consideration how LGBTQ-friendly their families are, what their socio-economic status is, what their local culture is like, whether they are a subsection of the LGBTQ that is sometimes misread as straight (bisexual people in cross-gender relationships and non-binary people in relationships that are read as heterosexual, for instance), and whether they have experienced other intersectional prejudices (due to race, national origin, disability, or religion, for instance). LGBTQ people aren't generally given oppression scores at queer group meetings to judge whether they've suffered enough to need support. Chances are, if they're seeking out community support, they have some personal reason for doing so. The same goes for asexual people who might feel a connection with queer communities.

And finally, when asexual people want to participate in queer spaces, they are not there entirely to use those communities for resources and support. They can also provide them. Asexual people bring insight into romantic identity and breakdowns of different types of intimacy that aren't commonly discussed, especially if a queer space is very sex-focused. Many non-asexual queer people who have engaged with asexual communities have learned about sophisticated models of attraction that were useful to them in their own non-normative relationships, and some are surprised to learn how much asexual people can contribute to queer discussion and moral support when given the chance.

Asexual people can provide insight on how to have relationships with asexual partners, and they can enrich the discussion with specialized, nuanced vocabulary that may be useful to queer folks too. And since many queer groups are becoming more asexual-friendly, many individual non-asexual queer folks welcome the chance to access informed understandings of how to be good asexual allies and how to support asexual people in their organizations.

On queer people limiting access to their space for LGBT issues only:

Regardless of whether they identify with queerness, asexual people do need to recognize that if they are heteroromantic or aromantic, they may be seen as a reminder of straightness; when queer people create their own space, they sometimes don't like to feel that someone they count as straight (or benefits from heterosexual privilege) is in it.

There is much evidence of a need for a "safe space," and people who don't identify as LGBT are far more likely to be coming from a position of ignorance and may behave/speak/dominate in ways that heterosexual people tend to do. In short, LGBT people want to have a space where what they hear from the heterosexual world all the time is not going to come up when they're in this supportive atmosphere. **Some LGBT folks feel unsafe discussing their issues in the presence of people who haven't experienced them or couldn't experience them.**

Heteroromantic and aromantic asexual people must recognize that many of them are afforded some modicum of heterosexual privilege—an argument that also comes up often when gay people discuss bisexual, polysexual,[19] and

---

19 *Polysexual* refers to someone who is sexually attracted to people of multiple sexes and genders, but not all sexes and genders. It is not the same as someone who is in sexual or romantic relationships with multiple people.

pansexual[20] people, who might be seen as straight by society part of the time depending on whether their relationships happen to be cross-gender (or perceived that way) at the time. A heteroromantic or aromantic asexual person—or pretty much anyone who passes as straight—could be seen as a reminder of the people who have attacked the queer people looking for relief. Regardless of whether a heteroromantic or aromantic asexual person feels queer, the outside world often sorts them into the straight box (however uncomfortably), and **not being sorted into the straight box comes with loss of safety, loss of comfort, and loss of privileges.**

And like many privileged people, most people experiencing heterosexual privilege have to be trained before they notice what it's done for them. Some LGBTQ people who more regularly experience oppression because of their orientation or gender presentation may bristle at the thought of people who have (presumably) never been attacked over their relationships choosing to identify as queer, especially if there is a perception that certain asexual people can belong with queer OR non-queer populations depending on their choice.

Some queer people may find asexual people particularly hard to be around because some mainstream narratives tell gay, lesbian, bisexual, polysexual, pansexual, transgender, non-binary, and gender-nonconforming people they should be celibate or not embrace their identity as a way to "save" themselves. It can be hard for a person who's been through conditioning to change or ignore their desires and identity to turn around and accept a person who does not have those desires (even though asexual people are often asked to go against *their* desires too).

There is a lingering pain that comes with some people's LGBT identity, especially in a society that has shamed their desires and forced them to fight for an opportunity to declare pride. Some of this shame can be deeply internalized, even if it's overcome in practice (and mostly so in attitude). LGBT people may believe the asexual people who want their support have never fought this type of shame and may not accept that "your orientation doesn't exist" can be as damaging as "your orientation means you're bad." Asexual people are usually perceived as sexually conservative or sexually abstinent, and LGBT people may have been attacked for the sex they may desire, so it could be very difficult for them to accept that someone who embodies a supposedly "ideal state" they've been pressured to emulate could possibly have comparable problems in Western society.

---

20 *Pansexual* refers to someone who is sexually attracted to people of all sexes and genders.

Most heteronormative cultures look at people as though they are straight until proven gay, and even asexual people (as long as they're in a hetero relationship or in no relationship) aren't likely to get stuck with the stigma many people with same-sex or same-gender partners have to deal with unless they choose to share the details. And while most queer people do not *define* the experience of queerness primarily around the amount or type of oppression they experience, it is undeniable that a certain alienation, instilled shame, and institutionalized persecution is often part of the LGBT package deal. In a world in which *queer* can be used as a slur, people who are electing to embrace it when it seems like they've never had it branded on their foreheads may be believed to want community and "specialness" without the hard knocks that go with it.

If someone is asexual and does not have these experiences but still wants the fellowship and community of queer folks, they should not be surprised if some insiders may automatically see them as interlopers. As asexual people, they have their own difficulties, but LGBT people who do not support asexual inclusion often believe that asexual people's difficulties aren't *their* difficulties (unless they also have a same-sex-oriented and/or trans identity).

So, if asexual people encounter resistance when asking queer people to acknowledge them, they should try to realize that queer folks may feel the asexual people are not respecting their identity. Asexual people should acknowledge that they haven't been through what LGBT people have been through (unless they have, as a person with another LGBTQ identity in addition to asexuality). They should be aware that their experience, while possibly also oppressive, probably also prejudicial, and definitely sometimes uncomfortable, isn't the same, and LGBT people may feel queer communities *are* only for those who do have those specific experiences (or have the capacity to).

Non-LGBT asexual people who want to network with and be included in LGBTQ groups may be more readily accepted if they demonstrate what they can give to their queer community instead of emphasizing what they need or want from it. They can learn to be listeners and apologize when they get it wrong. They can educate themselves on queer issues and support LGBT causes vocally and through action. They can make an effort to expose themselves to queer media (movies, television, and books with LGBT themes) and participate with LGBT friends at queer-centered social events, fundraisers, and pride demonstrations. They can follow their queer peers' lead in activist matters to the extent that they are welcome. And they can call out homophobia and transphobia in their own communities. Belonging may or may not come in time, but if a non-LGBT asexual person truly wants to ally with queer communities, they'll support them even if they aren't explicitly rewarded and included.

When in doubt, asexual people shouldn't accept that LGBT people are the gatekeepers on who can feel "queer," but they shouldn't attack LGBT people's desire to control access to their spaces. That's where their needs may be perceived as overstepping boundaries, and they shouldn't make everything about their issues unless their thoughts are welcome. If unsure, an asexual person who does not want to risk intruding or making anyone uncomfortable may at first choose to attend only those groups and events that are also open to allies and request inclusion in other queer events and spaces if everyone involved is comfortable.

On queerness itself:

Queer is pretty subjective—both for the people dictating who can be recognized as queer and for those identifying that way. *Queer* is usually considered an umbrella term. In its broadest sense, *queer* is said to be any form of gender identity/expression or sexual identity that is outside the norm. Some of the following might—but not necessarily do—identify as queer: those who are not heterosexual; those who are agender, between-gender, bigender, non-binary, third-gender, neutrois, or gender-shifting; those who are transgender;[21] and those who are kinky or polyamorous.

And though *queer* can be a controversial term because it's also used as an insult sometimes, most queer people of various stripes feel it is a positive word since its reclamation. But since it's so broad, meaning different things to different people, it's difficult to define "what is queer." Therefore, there is no dependable litmus test by which to determine what *isn't*. The queer movement itself stands for rejection of overly strict definitions that limit people's options in life, so some say it's counterintuitive to draw lines that exclude only certain types of less typical sexual, romantic, and gender identities and orientations.

Labels are tools we use to communicate with each other. Deciding whether to identify with the word *queer*—or whether to agree with someone else's identification as queer—may really be more about deciding whether *queer* necessitates homosexuality or non-cis gender, or whether it can also mean "not heteronormative." Most people recognize they should respect another person's labels and methods of self-identifying regardless of their personal definitions.

---

21 Some folks prefer the term *transsexual*, but it is often considered offensive or rude. When in doubt, use *transgender*, but if someone identifies as transsexual, that's their right.

Some asexual people *don't* feel they are queer and prefer to specifically identify as the asexual-spectrum label that describes them. Some just don't find it useful to be vaguer by saying "queer." But those who don't identify as queer might still be interested in allying

> "I do *not* think of myself as straight and will correct the impression when appropriate, but it describes well enough the way I'm treated by society, so I can't logically claim to understand what it's like to have all my social interactions—including family, to whom I haven't even needed to come out— colored by my orientation. While 'straight' does not describe me, neither does 'queer,' and I would assume most people who claim that label have their reasons for it."
>
> —REBECCA

with LGBTQ communities, and these communities may benefit from including information about and support for asexual people in their materials and events. More resources that can be incorporated into queer libraries and organizations are available in Part Six, the resources section of this book.

"Do You Consider Yourself Part of the LGBT Community?"

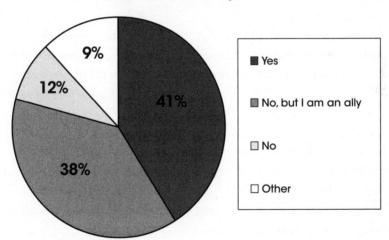

Reported in one survey of self-identified asexual-spectrum people collected on the Internet September–October 2011[22]

"Asexual" isn't another name for a heterosexual person who hates or avoids sex. **Asexual people are also fighting for recognition and tolerance,**

22 Community Census. (Asexual Awareness Week, 2011)

just like LGBT people are, and some feel a sense of belonging because of their experiences fighting the same or analogous battles. But ultimately, it's important for people who use the term to understand why they're using it and to be aware above all that it doesn't mean the same thing to everyone.

Some critics of the asexual awareness movement have opined that asexual people should not suggest they experience discrimination and should not present themselves as experiencing oppression. This opinion comes from heteronormative and queer populations alike, but seems especially vitriolic from some who feel their oppression is "real" while asexual people's is not. And sometimes, if an asexual person brings up something oppressive or discriminatory that has happened to them as a result of being asexual, they will often be told their unfortunate experience was *not* due to them being asexual. For example:

An aromantic asexual person gets misinterpreted as gay because he never couples up and gets beat up after school: "That wasn't anti-asexual violence. That was motivated by *gay* hatred, not asexual hatred."

A man sexually harasses an asexual woman and claims he can "fix" her, and eventually sexually assaults her because he thinks he's going to "wake up" her sleeping sexual appetite: "That wasn't anti-asexual violence. That was motivated by *misogyny*, not asexual hatred."

Asexual people may become withdrawn from communicating with co-workers because they were alienated by pressure to disclose sexual exploits at work, and eventually they are fired for not being a team player: "That wasn't anti-asexual prejudice. That was motivated by *their failure to fit in the culture*, not asexual discrimination."

Et cetera.

Even if terrible things happen to asexual people directly because of their asexuality, their experience is often pawned off on another "real" cause, suggesting that asexual people's reports of problematic reactions to their asexuality are exaggerated or nonexistent, and if they happened at all, they're "anecdotal" and probably not worth considering as a consistent problem.

The consistency with which this happens is good evidence that a concerted effort to silence asexual voices *is* happening. **Asexual people's orientation is almost always considered the least relevant aspect of their identity, and therefore, it is rarely accepted as the cause of their negative experiences.** For instance, it is impossible to separate a gay woman's lesbianism from her being a woman, because she is both. If someone hates a gay woman for being a gay woman, you can't isolate those aspects of her and say she only receives that hate because of one or the other. Prejudice against asexual people does exist, and it does manifest in nasty ways, but it should *always* be understood in the context of the whole person. Aspects of identity are inextricably intersectional. There is no practical purpose in separating them and calculating which ones "deserve" more attention.

Eradicating misogyny and homophobia before even *considering* asexual-specific issues on the agenda is ridiculous—especially since the attitudes that perpetuate harassment against LGBTQ populations often sprout from the same heteronormative root and can often be fought through the same educational efforts (and sometimes through the same organizations).

The tools used to measure prejudice and discrimination cannot be molded to detect LGBTQ oppression and then get applied unchanged to detect it in asexual populations. The asexual population's disadvantages will not look the same on the outside. It would be like expecting asexual people to get "asexual-bashed" coming out of the asexual bar while ignoring that **there are no asexual bars**. Sometimes asexual people hear objections like "how dare you say you have significant problems—I don't see your marriage getting rejected" or "the worst thing you deal with is someone calling you frigid, while *I* can't legally adopt a child with my partner." These perspectives suggest asexual people aren't suffering if they don't suffer the same way, but anti-asexual prejudice doesn't deny them the same things in all cases. This would be like saying a person of any oppressed group isn't *really* suffering if they have enough to eat.

While institutional discrimination against asexual people is not as visible and not as common as the types of institutional discrimination gay, bisexual, polysexual, pansexual, non-binary, and trans people experience, asexual people *do* have the capacity to experience it, and it has been documented. Below is a short (and non-exhaustive) list of laws, situations, attitudes, and issues that can and do specifically target and negatively affect asexual people, followed by discussion of each:

1. Consummation laws
2. Adoption denial
3. Employment discrimination and housing discrimination
4. Discrimination by mental health professionals
5. Lack of marriage equivalent for non-romantic relationships
6. Religious pressure/discrimination
7. "Corrective" rape
8. Lack of representation in media and sex education
9. Internalized oppression/self-hate

Consummation laws: Some states, provinces, territories, and countries have laws that require "consummation" of a marriage for it to be considered binding. While failure to agree to sex does not in itself void a marriage in all these cases, in some places a partner *can* get a marriage voided if the other partner refuses sex or cannot perform (though this interestingly does *not* apply to infertility).[23] Sex being a supported-by-law *requirement* of access to a secure marriage if the other partner so chooses to invoke it discriminates against repulsed asexual people (along with anyone else who cannot—or does not want to—make sex part of their relationship).

This is especially relevant in international marriages wherein one person is allowed to stay in the country because of marriage to another person who is a citizen. If the couple decides against having sex in the relationship (regardless of whether they are asexual), this can work against them when being interviewed by immigration officials about their relationship. Ultimately, if they are not having sex, they are far more likely to be suspected of not having a "real" marriage, faking the relationship to allow an immigrant to stay in the country under false pretenses. These interviews *can* include intensely personal questions about a couple's sex life and other practices, and it is simply considered obvious that every married couple will be having sex if they're really married.

Adoption denial: Same-gender couples have been widely scrutinized and discriminated against if they are parents or wish to adopt children. Is there an analogous situation for asexual people? An anecdotal source says yes. Adoption denials were reported,[24] with the asexual couples in question having their marriages scoffed at by decision-makers and denied as legitimate, contributing to a negative decision on their adoption application.

Employment and housing discrimination: Is there institutional discrimination of this sort for asexual people? At the time of this writing, most employers are not aware that asexuality is possible; however, perception that a person is not a team player, is not part of the shared culture, or is not sufficiently

---

23 "For instance, in some states, nonconsummation of a marriage is a ground for voiding the marriage. Failure to consummate renders it voidable, however, not void; the exception that proves this rule is South Carolina, where nonconsummation can render a marriage void, but cohabitation suffices to prove consummation. In addition, consummation of a marriage seals the marriage off from some attempts to void it. And while fraud is not generally grounds for voiding a marriage, fraudulent intent 'not to consummate the marriage or not to have intercourse likely to produce progeny' can be. Also striking is the fact that many states make impotence a ground for annulment, whereas infertility is not an independent ground for annulment in any state (unless misrepresented or concealed), suggesting that sex *per se* matters more to marriage than reproduction." (Emens, 2014)

24 "There was a couple of cases which were really, really distressing of asexual couples who approached Social Services to adopt children and Social Services asked them 'How come you don't have children by yourselves,' and the couple said 'We are asexual.' And Social Services said 'Well this is not normal, if you are asexual, you are not fit to be married.'" (Cormier-Otaño, 2011)

well-adjusted can result in poor treatment in the workplace, lack of opportunity, or even employment terminations[25] directly in association with being asexual.

Not being married after a certain age or having no romantic life can signal to superiors and co-workers that asexual people are "weird" or "have something off" about them and can interfere with their job performance or employers' perception of it.[26]

If a person is judged as antisocial or creepy because their relationships with others are not typical, they can be rejected as candidates for jobs and housing situations. (This is also a problem for those with mental illnesses, and it's compounded for asexual people who also have mental illnesses.) People who don't have romantic relationships and people who don't do what they're "supposed to" within their romantic relationships are subjected to scrutiny, shaming, and shunning, sometimes for no other reason than their orientation.

Discrimination by mental health professionals: Asexual people can also experience discrimination in mental health contexts. Acquiring mental health services for issues unrelated to sex or relationships becomes complicated if the therapist fixates on asexuality and/or aromanticism as a symptom of another disorder or incorrectly diagnoses an asexual person as having a disorder *because* of their asexuality.

In the past, using the version of the *Diagnostic and Statistical Manual of Mental Disorders* that was current from 1994 through 2013 (version IV), a diagnosis of "hypoactive sexual desire disorder" could be made based partly on whether a person's *partner* was distressed by their lack of interest in sex, even if they themselves were not distressed.[27] Now, under the latest diagnostic criteria as of this writing, both female sexual interest/arousal disorder[28] and male hypoactive sexual desire disorder[29] mention an exception for asexuality, claiming "If a lifelong lack of sexual desire is better explained by one's self-identification as 'asexual,'

---

25 In a blog post about the experience of getting fired from a job due to alienation over explicit sex talk in the work place, asexual employee Lasciel said, "I don't think I would have been fired if it hadn't been for my asexuality. The reason I was fired may have stemmed from a facet of my asexuality."

26 "A sexual minority bias was evident, whereby participants were most willing to rent to and/or hire heterosexuals relative to homosexuals, bisexuals, or asexuals." (MacInnis & Hodson, 2012)

27 Hypoactive Sexual Desire Disorder: "A. Persistently or recurrently deficient (or absent) sexual fantasies and desire for sexual activity. The judgment of deficiency or absence is made by the clinician, taking into account factors that affect sexual functioning, such as age and the context of the person's life. B. The disturbance causes marked distress or interpersonal difficulty. C. The sexual dysfunction is not better accounted for by another Axis I disorder (except another Sexual Dysfunction) and is not due exclusively to the direct physiological effects of a substance (e.g., a drug of abuse, a medication) or a general medical condition." (American Psychiatric Association, 2000)

28 "Lack of, or significantly reduced, sexual interest/arousal." (American Psychiatric Association, 2013)

29 "Persistently or recurrently deficient (or absent) sexual/erotic thoughts or fantasies and desire for sexual activity." (American Psychiatric Association, 2013)

then a diagnosis of female sexual interest/arousal disorder would not be made"[30] and "If the man's low desire is explained by self-identification as an asexual, then a diagnosis of male hypoactive sexual desire disorder is not made."[31]

However, many medical and psychological professionals assume that sexual attraction, sexual desire, and sexual arousal are part of every person's healthy life experience and may or may not be operating on closely held personal assumptions or older criteria they take for granted.

Asexual people have found themselves prescribed sexual arousal drugs or testosterone shots, or they were misinterpreted as lonely and repressed based on lack of certain relationships in their lives or were assigned trauma and/or fear they do not suffer from. Mental health professionals are sometimes distracted by what they think is a red flag and do not responsibly address their asexual clients' therapy.

Unavailability of marriage equivalents: Aromantic asexual people are far more likely than any other romantic or sexual orientation to gravitate toward nonsexual but established relationships that may function in a "life partner" capacity despite not being romantic or sexual. People who wish to cement a same-gender platonic partnership that includes living together, running a household, and possibly even raising children are affected by the same laws that same-gender couples are anywhere that currently outlaws their legal marriage; without access to "civil unions" for non-romantic and/or nonsexual relationships, their access to the benefits of marriage is limited,[32] even though they may function for many intents and purposes like a married couple.

Religious pressure/discrimination: While many LGBTQ people have been subjected to hurtful attitudes and attacks because of religious beliefs that categorize non-heteronormative behavior as sinful, asexual people can also be hurt by religious

"Depending on the denomination, the responses I have often received upon broaching the topic of asexuality range from the old-school 'it's an unnatural defiance of God's will' to the more psychologically-informed 'it's an unhealthy aversion.' (. . .) When it comes down to it, all of these statements make it clear that sexual attraction/desire is normalized as a characteristic of being human, and not experiencing it makes one just that little bit inhuman."

—M. LeClerc, *Hypomnemata*

---

30 Female Sexual Interest/Arousal Disorder. (American Psychiatric Association, 2013)

31 Male Hypoactive Sexual Desire Disorder. (American Psychiatric Association, 2013)

32 "Current regulation of sex devalues both sexual relationships that lack an intimate component and intimate relationships that lack a sexual component." (Rosenbury & Rothman, 2010)

attitudes. Though it is commonly assumed that asexual people would be supported by any religious individual or organization because they are perceived to be "pure" through abstinence, they do also run into harassment to date and mate as per the prescription to "be fruitful and multiply." If an asexual person lacks the urges that encourage reproduction, they can be deemed ungodly, unnatural, or going against their religious duty. Failure to reproduce is rarely regarded as a sin in and of itself, but failure to *try* to reproduce (presumably only when married) is not widely accepted by those following a religious agenda unless it is part of a vow one makes as clergy. Sexual expectations within marriage also affect married asexual people, and they may feel they have no choice—which is abusive.

"Corrective" rape: Asexual people are at a higher risk for "corrective" rape. Sometimes this is because they are commonly interpreted as being a challenge for an aggressive, confident person to "turn." Other times this happens because a rapist feels that sex is very important for everyone and they really believe forcing someone into sex will wake them up. Disturbingly, these hypothetical rapists aren't necessarily strangers or acquaintances. Many times they are the asexual person's partner or spouse. Sex is presented as a given in romantic or partnered relationships, and while many recognize the appeal of "waiting for the right time," most do not acknowledge that some people just plain never want to make sex part of the relationship. Some believe sex is owed to them as part of their relationships and that they must coax their partners into having sex and bully them into accepting it.

This sounds horrible, but anyone who's ever discussed this issue in a public place will very quickly see comments defending the rapists and **insisting that the only abusive person in this relationship is the one withholding sex**. Since this is the common narrative in our society—that sex is part of the package deal—asexual people who do not desire sex in their relationships are often bullied into believing they have to have sex to deserve a relationship.

Lack of representation in media and sex education: With few or no examples of people like them in media and no mention of asexuality in sex ed, asexual people lack resources and context for their orientation. If everywhere they turn, they see a picture of maturity that only includes sexual relationships and sexual attraction, they may experience any number of negative consequences, from confusion and anxiety to depression and self-destructive behaviors.

Internalized oppression and self-hate: Given all the above, it's not uncommon for asexual people to follow the example everyone has set: to hate and fear the signs of asexuality and try to cover them up or erase them. The pervasive mocking of virginity, the emasculation and harassment of men who don't define themselves through sexual conquests, the degrading and defeminizing slurs lobbed at women who don't desire sex, and the association of asexual people with aliens and robots and lack of vitality can all lead to shame and fear. Asexual people may feel they are disgusting or inhuman and may feel forced to hide their real orientation behind denial, lies, or hypersexual behavior.

Finally, even if asexual people have never experienced violent attacks, institutional denial of rights, or widespread hostile attitudes, erasure and invisibility can still be markedly harmful to asexual individuals and asexual communities. "Shut up, you're not being hurt" is a pretty egregious example of erasure, incidentally.

In the late 1980s, Peggy McIntosh wrote a groundbreaking "privilege checklist"[33] that discussed the items in her "invisible knapsack," which she carries around perpetually due to the fact that she is white. She "unpacked" some of those items by showing her readers what she can take for granted as a white person in a predominantly white society.

This list was eagerly adapted by other groups, and now a widely circulated checklist exists to outline what comes with heterosexual privilege. But does a phenomenon exist that uniquely oppresses asexual people, or are asexual people lumped in with all non-normative sexualities (or assumed heterosexual)? In other words, does something like "sexual privilege" exist that can benefit queer-sexual people as well as heterosexual people?

Some asexual people have considered whether "sexual privilege" exists, and the consensus is that "privilege" is the wrong word even though being asexual can be disadvantageous in society. Most just say there is definite prejudice and unpleasantness, but not in such a way that it would be classified as oppression. Ultimately, for sexual privilege to exist, it would mean that people who experience sexual attraction and feel included by the sexual culture would be offered advantages denied to people who do not in a systematic way that benefits the majority.

While the possibility of prejudice toward asexual people based entirely on their orientation has been examined,[34] some will say asexual invisibility

---

33 This concept was examined in McIntosh's "White Privilege: Unpacking the Invisible Knapsack." (McIntosh, 1989)

34 "[W]e uncovered strikingly strong bias against asexuals in both university and community samples. Relative to heterosexuals, and even relative to homosexuals and bisexuals, heterosexuals: (a) expressed more negative attitudes toward asexuals (i.e., prejudice); (b) desired less contact with asexuals; and (c) were less willing to rent an apartment to (or hire) an asexual applicant (i.e., discrimination)." (MacInnis & Hodson, 2012)

protects asexual people, leaving cisgender heteroromantic and aromantic asexual people to receive heterosexual privilege as a matter of course unless they go out of their way to tell those with power over them that they are asexual. But as we can see if we unpack, some of those givens are not actually in the asexual knapsack, indicating at least some experience of exclusion from participation as a full member of society.

Most people who experience sexual attraction (or experience/express sexual attraction normatively) don't realize how asexual people are excluded from the opportunities and lifestyle they may take for granted. *Privilege* isn't the right word, but let's at least assume for purposes of this discussion that **being a person who experiences sexual attraction can be (and usually is) advantageous in Western society, when contrasted with the experiences of those who don't**. Here are some experiences and concepts most people take for granted, but that exclude asexual people:

- Plenty of movies, television shows, documentaries, and fictional media feature characters who have feelings of sexual attraction, and said media acknowledges that these people exist (fostering information about and comfort with sexual attraction).
- Feeling sexual attraction or interest isn't considered a treatable mental illness by mainstream mental health professionals.
- Various sexual orientations that involve sexual attraction have been examined in physical, psychological, and social studies, resulting in a wealth of academic data on these groups.
- If asked to check a box representing their sexual orientation, there are generally a series of boxes for various types of people who feel sexual attraction and interest.
- Many people who experience sexual attraction were aware that their sexual orientation was an option before they reached puberty, and they were given the context to understand that others felt the same way they did.
- Physical organizations, help lines, and dedicated therapists exist that specifically offer help for issues that folks who experience sexual attraction might have with their sexuality or problems that arise from expressing it.
- People who experience sexual attraction are not told that they are aliens, seen as passionless, or assumed to be frigid based on their sexual orientation.[35]

---

35 "Asexuals were attributed significantly lower uniquely human traits than any other sexual orientation group." (MacInnis & Hodson, 2012)

- Possible partners of various sexual orientations who experience sexual attraction are at least fairly plentiful.
- If they have to discuss their sexuality or disclose it to someone, those who experience sexual attraction don't get called to defend that it exists.
- People with a capacity for sexual attraction are not frequently misinterpreted as being religious when they disclose their sexual orientation.
- People who are sexually attracted to each other can call their relationship romantic without frequent challenges to the relationship's legitimacy.
- Literature assumes that romantic relationships will be sexual when they are serious or committed enough, and this is an assumption that accurately reflects the experience of people who feel sexual attraction or interest.
- People who experience sexual attraction and interest are not assumed to be ignorant about sex or put off by discussions or images of sex because of their sexual orientation.

And here are some experiences and concepts that exclude or potentially exclude LGBT people. Every one of these also excludes asexual people.

- Commercials generally present sexually motivated advertising that is appropriate for cisgender heterosexual people.
- Cis heterosexual people don't get asked to give the cis and hetero community's perspective or consensus on issues. Cis and heterosexual people are not seen as representatives of all people of the same orientation/identity.
- Cis heterosexual people are not told that their identity or orientation will change once they meet the right person.
- Heterosexual people's sexual orientation isn't generally used as an insult. Cisgender people's gender identity is not generally used as an insult.
- Cis heterosexual people's gender identity and sexual orientation don't inspire anyone to wonder what their parents did wrong.
- Cis heterosexual people are not asked how their genitalia works or if their genitalia functions properly in response to declaring their identity or sexual orientation.
- Cis heterosexual people are not repeatedly told to have sex with people they're not attracted to so they can be "sure."
- Cis heterosexual people's identity and sexual orientation isn't commonly misinterpreted as hatred of another gender.
- Cis heterosexual people can enter a relationship without causing friends and loved ones to pity their partners on the basis of their gender identity and/or sexual orientation.

- Cis heterosexual people aren't generally told that their gender identity and sexual orientation will lead to them dying alone.
- Details of cisgender heterosexual people's masturbation habits aren't requested by strangers upon revealing one's identity and orientation, and these details, if offered, aren't used against them to assign them denial or a disorder.
- Doctors acknowledge that heterosexual attraction exists and is healthy and do not assume those who claim to experience it are hiding information or lying.
- Feeling heterosexual attraction does not inspire loved ones to insist that one get psychological and physical examinations before accepting one's sexuality.
- It's easy to get a group together consisting of people who are all cis and heterosexual.
- In polite conversation, it is not socially acceptable for others to tell cis heterosexual people that if they shared the same identity and orientation, it would make them want to die, commit suicide, "go crazy," or "get help."
- Cis heterosexual people are not frequently misinterpreted as "going through a phase," "mentally immature," or "physically immature" because of their orientation/identity.
- Cis heterosexual people are not told that they're not "real" representatives of their gender based on their sexual orientation.
- Cis heterosexual people are not regularly described as "broken" or "needing to be fixed" if they are honest regarding their identity and attraction experiences.
- If they need therapy, cis heterosexual people's gender identity and/or sexual orientation isn't likely to be invoked as either a symptom or a cause of any disorders or problems they have.
- Cis heterosexual people aren't asked why they're cisgender and heterosexual or how/when they got that way.
- Cis heterosexual people can casually call attention to their gender identity or mention their relationships without others accusing them of creating an uncomfortable situation.
- Cis heterosexual people do not face automatic assumptions that they will not have children because of their gender and orientation.
- Cis heterosexual people don't have to "come out" to be honest.
- Cis heterosexual people rarely have to be in a situation in which they are the only cisgender heterosexual person in the room.

- No one thinks being cisgender or heterosexual is only likely as the result of abuse.
- Most leaders and authority figures and role models will be cis heterosexual people.

So clearly, moving through the world as an asexual person does put one at a disadvantage, and asexual people share quite a few of these experiences with those in queer communities. Also, people who are not affected personally have a tendency to underestimate the effect these disadvantages have on people who live this existence day in and day out. **It's very easy as someone who is not in the affected population to say "I see how my oppression affects me, but I don't believe yours is affecting you because it is irrelevant and invisible to me, so I refuse to consider that it is real."** There are far too many parallels here to claim asexual people as a group do not experience prejudice and cannot be hurt by it.

Invisibility means not being able to connect with others like you. It means being very likely to come to the conclusion that you are broken. It means seeing no boxes to check and being filled with fear or shame or frustration. It means being isolated in a way that is unimaginable to most people who take their visibility for granted. And it means that as soon as you try to *be* seen—regardless of whether you're just asking the initial questions or deliberately spreading asexual-specific awareness—the vile attitudes and unreasonable requests for justification you will be subjected to will probably make you wonder if that invisibility was really so bad.

Some LGBT people may have some inkling of what this kind of invisibility feels like if they have been forced to hide their identity and/or orientation for their whole lives or grew up in a time or place when *nobody* talked about what they were experiencing, but by and large LGBT issues are now acknowledged far and wide and asexual issues are still usually swept under the rug.

Any asexual person who identifies openly as asexual learns to defend the very existence of the orientation against comments like "No, see a head doctor" and "I'm sorry, but that's not a real thing" and "If you love someone, you have to want to have sex with them" and "Sex with me will fix you." Asexual people are told, through these messages, that they are expected to be quiet unless they *want* people to interrogate them about everything from sexual experiences to genital functionality.

Asexual people are commonly told they're only getting harassed because they disclosed their orientation—that they will only experience these discriminatory and prejudicial attitudes if they discuss it. Why, after all, would they bring it up if *not* bringing it up would free them from being criticized?

The above attitude is more or less advocating asexual people staying in the closet. That it's coming out itself that causes the problem, not any kind of issue with the mainstream attitude. If someone's "solution" to asexual prejudice and discrimination is to tell asexual people to keep their orientation a secret, they're saying the best solution to harassment is to lie by omission or pretend to be heterosexual. This is not a suggestion we see being made by LGBT allies for the most part; most truly supportive allies agree that if you're unable to publicly identify as your sexual orientation or gender identity, you're living in an oppressive atmosphere. It's not different for asexual people. They're not alone among all the sexual orientations as the one group that would be better off shutting their mouths or disclosing it only to potential partners.

And the messages asexual people are complaining about aren't along the lines of "Sometimes people say hurtful things to us." The messages are often much more subtle, and asexual people all grow up in the thick of them, building their brains around a "way things are" that doesn't fit them. Asexual people are not the only people this happens to. But when asexual people's problems are considered irrelevant even when they're brought out into the open, it's hard to imagine a much clearer example of invisibility than that.

Asexual Community

Asexual communities are very diverse places, but the intersection of the members' asexuality and their other circumstances is often unique. Here are some important concepts that are relevant in various asexual communities and some intersectional experiences of certain groups.

Young and Asexual

Because of asexual people's isolation by geography, much of the asexual conversation, connection, and communion is happening among a rather young crowd over the Internet. Because of this—and because young people typically discuss their identity with their peers more than older people do—the Internet-based asexual communities are getting more attention and being assumed more representative of the asexual population in general, which sometimes results in misleading information. For instance, young asexual people are overrepresented in polls, sometimes skewing the statistics and making outsiders less likely to take the orientation seriously because of a tendency to write off movements by young people as a phase. (This is problematic in its own right, but it happens to any movement whose membership is overwhelmingly young.) But contrary to some detractors' beliefs, the asexual culture is not entirely made up of college students.

Young asexual people, especially teens, deal with alienation and confusion when the media constantly portrays people their age as being hormonally driven or obsessed with sex and relationships—especially since their non-asexual peers will be developing their sexual attractions and are able to relate to said media. Asexual teens often feel frustrated by advertising and magazines that assume sexual attraction is part of their lives.

Young asexual people frequently face condescending and dismissive statements about their age, often from older adults (especially their parents), and sometimes even from their peers, who insist one day they'll develop sexual attraction when they mature or after they have sex. However, since most people figure out by their early teens what kind of people they're attracted to, it makes sense that asexual people would feel asexual in their teens as well. Even though it's true that they may choose a different label later in life—as anyone might—and may find their tastes changing as they age, that doesn't mean there aren't asexual thirteen-year-olds out there. There are certainly heterosexual thirteen-year-olds and LGBTQ thirteen-year-olds!

Asexuality may look like a blank or a "not yet" when it describes a young teen, but keep in mind that if someone is asexual later in life, they probably already felt that way at this age.

Older and Asexual

The desexualization of older people starts fairly young. Kids like to pretend their parents don't have sex, and young people will scream "Gross!" if anyone with wrinkles engages in public displays of affection. It sends the clear message that adults ranging from midlife to senior citizens are *expected* to be sexless creatures. But are they in reality? Of course not.

There's a pervasive perception among the young that living a sexless life is in fact preferable and expected for elderly people. In reality, having a sex life is typical for people of all ages, and it is in fact unusual to be an older person with no sexual attraction to anyone. Older people who identify as asexual are often dismissed by younger people with phrases like "that's just how it is when you're older," even if the older asexual person never felt any interest when they were younger either.

How young can you be and still be old? When it comes to sex and relationships, age thirty seems to be an arbitrary number by which most people are expected to carve out their romantic life and make their family decisions. If someone has made such a decision and it involves choosing no one, they are usually assumed

to be undecided, search-
ing, desperate, hoping,
or stunted. Aromantic
asexual people who en-
ter later adulthood while
single deal with this misconception constantly.
Even those who say "I
like being single" will be
doubted and treated like
they're trying to cover

"Asexual people—usually women—who are in
their thirties still report being told that they're 'too
young' to know their sexual orientation, or that
they're just 'late bloomers.' The fact that asexuals
from this same age group are also told that
they're too old to have a sexuality, that their lack
of sexual attraction is simply what happens to
people in their thirties, shows that the point is to
invalidate asexuality by any means necessary."
—AYDAN SELBY, *MUSINGS OF AN IST*

shame for their failures. Partnered relationships are so expected in our society
that being happy without one is often regarded as impossible.

As for partnered asexual people who are older, many of them will have
spent the majority of their adult lives not knowing asexuality exists and making
a lot more compromises in their relationships with non-asexual partners than
they might have if they'd known. Many asexual people who are in relationships
without knowing they're asexual have accepted that sex is expected of them,
and they believe not being sexually attracted to their partners is just not something that should get talked about.

As awareness about asexuality grows, many partnered older asexual people
are realizing they internalized damaging ideas and accepted frustrating situations in the interest of staying partnered. They can have healthier relationships
if they include their partners in their revelations about themselves and negotiate
better compromises. And those older asexual people who are not partnered but
wish to be may be able to pursue partners more constructively than they did in
the past once they are armed with more knowledge about successful asexual
relationships. (Additional discussions of asexual relationships are offered in Part
Four and Part Five of this book.)

Older asexual people who were married and had families before discovering
their orientation may have the decidedly frustrating experience of coming out
not only to their spouses, but also to their kids. A child coming out to a parent
usually feels more risky since the parent has power over the child, but a parent
coming out to their child could make the child feel their parent is naive about
sex-related issues that matter to them or that they aren't really a respectable
adult. These are damaging (and untrue) assumptions that can hurt families if the
children aren't receptive to the idea. That said, awareness is growing among the
younger generations, and this may be a smaller problem in the future.

However, older asexual people without partners are saddled with much more criticism and confusion than their partnered counterparts. If someone is single and they move past their twenties without "settling down," they are likely to be targeted with concern and sometimes unsolicited intervention even if they want to be single. Many asexual people who do not desire a partner find themselves frustrated with how often singlehood in one's late twenties and beyond is interpreted as pathetic or lonely, and many of them may internalize these accusations and find themselves adopting poor coping mechanisms and destructive behaviors in a world that seems to have no place for someone like them.

Older men who are not married are usually excused more readily; women in their thirties and beyond are often regarded with pity, regarded as "no longer young" and therefore less valuable, and assumed unwanted and unlovable. Conversely, men who aren't married at that age are usually assumed to have chosen to be so or to be "career focused" (unless they fall into certain perceived-to-be-undesirable categories, such as being aesthetically unappealing or effeminate; in those cases they may also be regarded as sad people who are single because no one would choose them).

Regardless of how they act or what they say or do, partnerless women past thirty are perceived as lonely "cat ladies" or as desperate for men (or regarded as creepy and "on the prowl"), and may be called condescending, sexualized, or misleading names (*old maid* or *spinster* if they seem uninterested in partners, *MILF* or *cougar* if they do want a partner)—and none of these terms have analogous male equivalents that don't apply to younger men too. Misunderstandings about midlife sex-drive peaks and menopausal hormones may lead some people to think partnerless asexual women will inevitably "blossom" during a supposed sexual prime.

Not being married or partnered—especially for women—is perceived as practically pathological, and society tends to process partnerless people as either desperate to change their status or as resigned to a sad life. When people are younger and partnerless, they're usually considered "not married *yet*," while older people are frequently asked, "*why* aren't you married?" or "*when* are you going to find a mate and have some kids?" Partnered, family-oriented life is regarded as the default—as something we can assume everyone wants, and we're certainly considered a failure if we haven't achieved it by our third decade. This issue disproportionately affects older asexual people who either don't want a partner or have trouble finding one who won't regard their asexuality as "a sex problem."

However, we don't know as much about the attitudes and experiences of the pre-Internet generation of asexual people because most of the census data is gathered through Internet communities whose populations skew young, leaving the voices of older asexual people underrepresented. As more awareness spreads, more older asexual people will recognize themselves in the description, and as the generation that spurred widespread use of the term *asexual* ages, fewer tropes like "this is a phase for the young" will persist in popular perceptions of asexual people.

Asexual Women, Asexual Men

There are more women than men represented in asexual communities.[36] The reasons for this are not completely clear since asexual people as a group have not been subjected to much scientific study, but certain gender-specific trends hint at some possible reasons.

First of all, there aren't as many men online or in meetup groups talking frankly about feelings or lack of feelings, so in some cases men may simply be less inclined to participate in asexual communities. Also, many people believe men have higher sex drives, which may contribute somewhat to their seeking out sex even without attraction. They may be less likely to recognize anything different about how/why they seek out sex, especially since men aren't as likely to be shamed for avoiding committed partnership or emotional attraction while still desiring sexual activity. If they're sexually functional cisgender men, they may believe their ability to get erections and their response to stimuli means they can't be asexual or that they must be sexually attracted to anyone with whom they enjoy sexual activities.

Men are also popularly expected to define themselves through sexual conquests, lust, and bedroom performance, so sometimes they can be less likely to identify as asexual because they fear having their masculinity challenged. Also, more asexual men report being willing to have sex they don't particularly want when pressured or invited; among men, sex is usually considered less of a "big deal" to try despite lack of interest, though there are, of course, asexual men who are sex repulsed. They may be shamed by partners if they do not desire their partners sexually, and they may be invalidated by outside observers if they have partners with whom they do not have sex.

Heteronormative men are also more likely to label other men homosexual, as failures who "can't get laid," or as having "just given up" if they aren't aggressive about chasing women, so this sort of peer pressure and the stigma some people associate with homosexuality can make it much harder to come out as an asexual man than it is to come out as an asexual woman.

---

36 During one survey administered over the Internet in September–October 2011, about 64 percent of those surveyed identified as female, with only about 14 percent identifying as male. (The rest were "other" or non-binary gender in some way.) (Asexual Awareness Week, 2011)

And among gay, bisexual, polysexual, and pansexual men, a man with same-gender romantic leanings but no sexual leanings may be treated like he is repressing his sexuality because of internalized oppression or shame. Queer men who don't pursue other men sexually or don't experience sexual attraction can be harassed to get past their supposed hangups, leaving them assuming their disinterest is a hurdle, not an orientation. It is possible that some combination of fewer asexual men existing and fewer asexual men realizing their orientation/coming out has resulted in men's lower numbers in asexual communities.

Some teenage boys may be able to shrug off the taunts and harassment they may receive when they aren't enraptured with pornographic magazines or constantly talking about which partners they would like to have sex with, but most are very alienated by it if they are unlucky enough to become targets. Girls, of course, also talk about desired partners, but in their younger years, girls may be more positively regarded (or at least not as often harassed) if they're not obsessed with sex. Not all boys are immersed in this culture, but most are aware of it and many are affected by it.

However, as people get older, men and women are expected, because of heteronormative assumptions, to define themselves through relationships with each other, and men are sometimes assumed weak and spineless if they haven't "gotten" a partner while women are assumed pathetic and lonely if no one has "chosen" them. Regardless of whether they want to date, marry, or have sex, they will be judged by these standards for not doing it if they choose not to and may feel pressure to behave normatively so they go against their own inclinations. Fostering knowledge about asexuality may help both of these genders minimize uncomfortable expectations.

Asexual People of Color

White asexual people are *very* overrepresented at all levels, especially Internet-based communities. Class and socioeconomic status are partially to blame for this in the West, because the Internet is less accessible to many non-white groups and in non-white-majority countries, and since asexual communities form and educate and congregate overwhelmingly on the Internet as of this writing, this tends to minimize the involvement of people of color. But there are many other roadblocks to people of color embracing an asexual orientation or identifying with asexual communities as well.

Asexual people of color are more invisible than white asexual people. Because people of color within Western culture are more criticized, more harshly observed, held to higher/different standards, and in general already viewed/treated as "other" in many societies, it can be very difficult to come out when doing so can result in rejection from one's own community or family.

First off, there's the problem of not feeling like part of an in-group

> "My asexuality doesn't save me from racism—it just means I get to deal with people being racist *and* anti-ace, sometimes simultaneously. Despite the thrilling arguments about asexuality being a 'white sexuality,' white supremacy doesn't want me to be asexual any more than the patriarchy does."
>
> —QUEENIE, *THE ASEXUAL AGENDA*

if they attempt to socialize in asexual spaces. Individual non-white asexual people have made great strides in asexual leadership and activism, but nearly all the mainstream news and visible asexual community efforts are fronted by white people, with the most popular communities dominated by white voices. Faced with an asexual community that is overwhelmingly white, asexual people of color may feel alienated and uncomfortable trying to find a place there, especially if the white majority talks over them or erases their experiences.

Some will join online asexual communities and not bring up their race as they perceive it may cost them a sense of belonging or because white participants may suggest their perspectives or discussions of race-related intersectionality are irrelevant. They may also feel pressured to consider class issues, race issues, and religious issues that affect their communities and cultures disproportionately as "more important" and may feel shamed for thinking attention to asexuality awareness is actually worthwhile.

There is also the fact that, from an early age, people of color—especially young black people and to some extent Hispanic and Latinx/Latino/Latina people—are automatically sexualized to a higher degree by white observers in Western society. Women in these groups are more often considered sexual objects (along with Asian women being fetishized), while black, Hispanic, and Latino men in these groups are regarded as overwhelmingly sexual. For these folks, being recognized as asexual and respected for it is markedly less likely, in some cases from both outside and inside their communities. They are assumed to like sex or be sexually promiscuous or have high sex drives more consistently than their white counterparts, and they can be defined by these interpretations in different ways both within and outside of their communities regardless of how they actually feel or behave.

Some asexual people of color are perceived as deliberately avoiding sex as some kind of commentary on or reaction to the "sensual, sexual" image thrust upon them, and may be regarded as rejecting their culture if they

> "By virtue of being black, I am already considered hypersexual by white society. That I am sexually attractive and I am sexually attracted to many people and act on those attractions regularly. By being an asexual who is not sexually attracted to anyone and is celibate, I can be seen as either combatting that racist stereotype or simply repressing my 'true sexuality' because of that racist stereotype."
>
> —FⅡSH

reject its supposed sexual norms. It can be perceived as simply a reaction rather than an organic expression of who they are.

And then there is the flip side: there are also cases of people of color being *desexualized* in certain situations; certain ethnicities are regarded by white outsiders as less sexual or prudish (like, in some cases, East/Southeast Asian people, especially men, or people of Middle Eastern descent, especially women). They're sometimes invalidated and told they're just repressing their instincts because their cultures have weird hangups about sex. Western society treats these groups as if they exist to perform certain functions for the majority rather than to have their own wants and needs, so their sexual agency is rarely respected.

If an asexual person of color comes out, they are sometimes assumed to be playing into these tropes rather than expressing their intrinsic lack of desire or attraction, and they may be subjected to attitudes like "well of course you're asexual, that's how people like you are" from the white majority and attitudes like "can you stop making us look like we're all frigid?" from within their own community. These folks may feel that all these messages mean asexuality is for white people and they are betraying their culture by buying into it.

And then there are certain non-white groups that value and enforce heteronormativity in such a way that people who don't conform (including LGBTQ and asexual people) may be treated like they are offending, disappointing, or bringing shame upon their community or family. Cultures wherein loyalty to the family unit is of utmost importance may expect sacrifice for the perceived good of the family and will not tolerate a person who comes out as asexual. They may interpret lack of conformity as a betrayal and may even threaten or go through with punishment and shunning. Coming out as asexual in these situations might cause unacceptable loss of access to family and community, which will disadvantage them more than a similar situation would disadvantage a white asexual person.

Being a minority within a minority requires safety, conviction, and comfort with one's environment that is not always available to the more persecuted and oppressed people in Western society. Asexuality will seem especially rare among racial minorities if the statistics are believed, but all signs point to their simply being less visible, and some of them face attitudes that are even less friendly to asexuality than the mainstream.

Gay / Queer and Asexual

Many asexual people consider themselves to be some form of LGB because their primary relationship is not a cross-gender relationship or is not perceived by others to be so. They may not specify that they are "asexual homoromantic" or "asexual panromantic" or whatever their full orientation is; if an asexual-identified person also calls themselves gay, bi, pan, or queer, they're usually referencing their romantic relationships or their patterns of romantic attraction.

Most asexual people tend to be supportive of consensual sexual relationships of any kind, including kink and polyamory. Acceptance is the norm in many asexual spaces online, and any kind of hate speech is frowned upon, though of course it still occurs (and isn't always dealt with appropriately). Not all asexual people support queer orientations, but since there is *lots* of overlap between asexuality and these other marginalized sexual and romantic minority groups as well as *lots* of opportunity for empathy, phobic attitudes are not generally tolerated.

Many asexual people who experience romantic attraction to their own gender and/or to more than one gender enjoy being part of queer communities, but they may find that their asexuality confuses or upsets other queer folks. They may be mistaken for suffering from internalized homophobia if they do not desire sex, do not experience sexual attraction, or are not willing to engage in sex. In these spaces, sometimes they're strongly encouraged to "get over" their supposed reluctance to have sex, and more education about asexuality in LGBTQ spaces can help avoid these harmful assumptions.

Transgender and Asexual

Transgender communities and asexual communities have a significant amount of overlap. There are transgender asexual people, and both groups seem to know more about each other's existence and issues than the general population—probably partly because of how much education both groups do on the Internet and the special efforts of trans asexual educators. There is no known cause-effect relationship between being asexual and being transgender, but on surveys and in online forums, the percentage of people identifying as transgender is higher than it is in the non-asexual population.

In a survey of 3,436 self-identified asexual-spectrum people administered on the Internet in September–October 2011, respondents were asked to state whether they considered themselves transgender[37]:	
Yes	10.2%
No	80.4%
Unsure	9.4%

* This survey was limited to one answer.

A fraction of trans people who plan to transition or are going through transition feel asexual only until they've begun transition or transitioned (possibly due to dysphoria), though most trans asexual people continue to identify as asexual in post-transition life.

Sometimes trans asexual people who wish to medically transition will be asked why they want to have surgery if they don't intend to have sex. This question is sometimes even offered by other transgender people and is usually presented as though the asexual trans person is unreasonable or behaving paradoxically. Putting aside that being asexual doesn't even necessarily mean a person won't have sex, a transgender person who wants a medical transition usually has many reasons besides using their genitalia for sex. Even if nobody except the transgender person in question ever saw them naked, having the genital configuration they want is very important for some. Not all transgender people feel surgery is necessary for transition, but those who do aren't necessarily doing it for reasons related to sexual intercourse.

Trans asexual people can find support and camaraderie in some asexual organizations and groups online.

Other Non-Cisgender / Non-Binary Identities and Asexuality

Acceptance of various non-normative, non-cisgender, and non-binary identities is common in asexual communities.

In a survey of 3,436 self-identified asexual-spectrum people administered on the Internet in September–October 2011, respondents gave the following answers when asked to provide their gender identity[38]:	
Female	64.1%
Male	14.1%
Gender neutral	12.0%

---

37 Community Census. (Asexual Awareness Week, 2011)
38 Community Census. (Asexual Awareness Week, 2011)

Androgynous	11.4%
Gender queer or gender variant	11.1%
Gender fluid	8.0%
Unsure/confused	7.5%
Questioning	6.6%
I don't have a gender identity	6.2%
Other	4.3%

* Participants were allowed to choose more than one answer

As seen in the gender census above, a significant portion of asexual people consider themselves gender neutral (or neutrois), androgynous, genderqueer, gender variant, gender fluid, unsure, questioning, without gender (or agender), or something else non-binary.

There is no known cause-effect relationship between being a non-binary gender and being asexual, but there is significant overlap in these populations. One's gender and one's attraction to others are, of course, related for most people, and not identifying as one of the most common genders may be tied up with complications in how one relates to others sexually and romantically, but that does not at all imply that being non-binary causes asexuality or vice versa.

In communities that encourage exploration of the self and help provide new perspectives on assumptions about gender and sexuality that many take for granted, it makes sense that more people would feel comfortable identifying as non-binary or would gravitate toward participating in communities that foster both their gender identity and their sexual orientation.

All non-binary identities will find similar people in asexual communities and can enjoy support from others like them, with whom they can discuss gender presentation and the intersection of their gender with their sexual orientation. Some non-binary folks call themselves *enby/enbies* (formed from saying the initials for non-binary—N.B.—out loud). And in asexual spaces online, some non-binary asexual people who needed a space to discuss gender issues began to refer to themselves as *transyadas*, and they created their own forum.[39]

Autistic and Asexual

Autistic communities and asexual communities also have an overlap.[40] There are commonalities between some autistic folks and some asexual people.

---

39 *Transyada* forum: transyada.net/forum/
40 "[A] higher rate of asexuality was found among individuals with [Autistic Spectrum Diagnoses]." (Gilmour & Schalomon, 2012)

For instance, some autistic people have atypical ways of forming relationships and emotional attachment, and it is much more common for an autistic person to be touch averse than for a non-autistic person to be so,[41] which may hinder some adult autistic people's ability to form romantic relationships (or at least may lower their confidence in attempting to do so). And some autistic people are on the other end of the spectrum, craving touch to maintain their well-being. Being cuddly and wanting tactile stimulation can be misinterpreted as sexual advances in some adult relationships, so asexual autistic people in this situation can experience high levels of frustration.

There has been no cause determined, no genetic or other type of link between asexuality and autism, but there is a correlation. However, most asexual people are not autistic, nor are most autistic people asexual. It's simply been noted that the percentage of known autistic people in the known asexual population is higher than that of the general population; some say it might be because both communities encourage self-analysis and self-examination, which leads to more people identifying non-normative traits about themselves. An autistic asexual person can find community and be in good company.

Unfortunately, a pervasive tendency to desexualize autistic people contributes to the perception that asexuality is *part of* autism or at least that if an autistic person does not pursue or desire sexual relationships, that it is directly because of their autism (or that if they do pursue such relationships, it's "in spite of" their autism). There are so many different kinds of autism, and so many different ways of forming asexual relationships, that it would be misleading to conflate asexuality and autism as necessarily intertwined with each other.

This narrative of ignoring the sexuality of autistic people can sometimes make asexual autistic people feel ashamed of coming out; they may worry their visibility might strengthen the belief that autistic people aren't sexually inclined or that asexual people are all autistic. But autistic people are a natural percentage of every population, and asexual communities are enriched by the neurodiversity they provide.

Some autistic asexual people believe their autism and their asexuality are not at all related to each other. Some other asexual autistic people do feel that the two are linked, but they usually say so only while speaking for themselves. This is a lead everyone who knows an asexual autistic person should follow.

---

41 In a study comparing typically developing children with children on the autistic spectrum, 22.1 percent of the autistic children "react emotionally or aggressively to touch" when compared with only 5 percent of typical children. (Tomchek & Dunn, 2007)

Disability, Illness, Mental Illness, Disorders, and Asexuality

Asexual people can have disabilities and illnesses—visible and invisible[42]—and can often experience higher than average harassment rates because of these complicating factors. Detractors perceive that they have a disability or a disorder or a condition, proceed to use it to invalidate their experience of themselves, and cause them stress. And just like other groups that experience discrimination, alienation, and hardship, asexual people may experience depression and substance abuse at a higher rate than the general population.[43] But it's well known in asexual communities that some cross-section of any population will have a disability, a health condition, a disorder, or a mental illness. Asexuality isn't an orientation that can only be claimed by those with able bodies and optimum health.

Asexual people are subjected to most or all of the same pressures in society as everyone else with their other traits, and they can suffer from self-image issues, eating disorders, social anxiety, and many other issues, regardless of whether or how much their orientation and related experience has to do with it. Sometimes disabilities and health conditions can affect or be related to lack of libido, lack of interest in sex, or lack of passion for or ability to engage in sex, but if this is the case for a person who self-describes as asexual, there is really no practical reason to say that person's experience of asexuality is less legitimate. Everyone is affected by their physical existence, and *asexual* is what we call someone who isn't experiencing sexual attraction to others, regardless of *why*.

Asexual people with disabilities or health issues are often told "you just feel that way because of your condition," as if that would make it less "real" or as if a sexual orientation could clearly have a single "cause." It'd be like saying to a non-asexual person, "You just want sex because your hormones are making you think you do." In other words, useless, demeaning, and pointlessly oversimplified. Most asexual communities understand and accept that people with disabilities and health issues do not have a less valid form of asexuality.

Asexual people and people with disabilities have one (problematic) thing in common: they are often regarded by outside populations as being less human,

---

42 Some "visible" disabilities and illnesses include symptoms or require use of equipment that can be seen, while "invisible" disabilities and illnesses will not be apparent unless they are disclosed; some invisible disabilities and illnesses include chronic pain, mental illnesses and mood disorders, sensory problems and sensory processing problems, medical problems controlled with medication or kept under control through diet and limited activity, and illnesses with long treatment plans like cancer.

43 "Large-scale studies on mental health issues in gay men and lesbian women have found evidence that these sexual minorities do have higher rates of mental health problems (e.g. depression, substance abuse) than heterosexual individuals. [. . .] If asexual people feel similar pressure to other sexual minorities to conform to heterosexual norms, then it is possible that they too may have elevated rates of mental health problems." (Yule, Brotto & Gorzalka, 2013)

less complete, "suffering" from their situation, or missing something. The conflation of disability with lack of sexuality is a big problem for everyone in both these groups, but especially so for people who are both asexual and have a disability. Not only is their asexuality written off as a symptom of their disability, but it helps reinforce people's belief that all people with disabilities are asexual (or at least that people with disabilities do not want or desire sex, do not experience arousal, or do not want partners).

It's very important to understand that asexuality can coexist with disability and/or all types of illnesses—and interact with those conditions as part of being a whole person—without assuming that one causes the other or that they always go together. Asexual people with disabilities or illnesses shouldn't have to worry that announcing their orientation will reflect poorly on the validity of asexuality.

Many asexual people with disabilities or illnesses worry that coming out will contribute to the desexualization of disabled/ill people or to the misconception that people become asexual because of disabilities or illnesses. Increased focus on the intersection of both can help prevent this. It would be ridiculous to suggest the asexual population, as large as it is, would contain no one with disabilities or illnesses, so why should those people be singled out and told their disability or illness is the most important aspect of who they are when it comes to how they experience attraction?

There's nothing wrong with suggesting that a disability or illness (or treatment for a condition) can and very well might interact with a person's experience of themselves in every way, including how they feel about potential partners. But an asexual person with a disability or illness isn't *just* one or the other, and it's not anyone's business to decide what conditions have to be fulfilled before a person's experience is designated as a symptom. It's all right for a person's asexuality to be partially tied into some aspect of their physical existence, and it's also all right for a person to say they *don't* believe their orientation has anything to do with a condition they have. Everyone is different in this regard. Most asexual people don't have disabilities or illnesses, and most people with them are not asexual, but where they intersect, there should still be respect for both.

Asexual People and Entertainment

Among Internet-savvy asexual folks, there is a wide appreciation for subcultures, but this shouldn't suggest that asexual people are by nature nerdy or socially awkward or that they are forced to be "geeks" because they can't have normal relationships.

Entertainment-wise, some asexual fans tend to appreciate television shows and other media works that center around characters who aren't consistently motivated by sex or are rumored to be asexual. Some examples at the time of this writing are the television shows *The Big Bang Theory*, *Sherlock*, and *Doctor Who*. Even though it's not necessary for a character to be "canon" asexual for asexual people to relate to them, it's also not completely unheard of for characters in fictional works to self-identify as asexual. Here are some examples of media containing explicitly asexual characters:

Television Shows:

Sirens (United States, USA Network, 2014 –) / Character: Voodoo
Divorce (The Netherlands, RTL 4, 2012 –) / Character: Desiree
Huge (United States, ABC Family, 2010) / Character: Poppy
Godiva's (Canada, Bravo!, 2005–2006) / Character: Martin
Shortland Street (New Zealand, Television New Zealand, 1992–) / Character: Gerald

Novels:

Demonosity (Amanda Ashby, Puffin, 2013) / Character: Nash
Quicksilver (R.J. Anderson, Carolrhoda Books, 2013) / Character: Tori
Banner of the Damned (Sherwood Smith, DAW, 2012) / Character: Emras
Guardian of the Dead (Karen Healey, Little, Brown, 2010) / Character: Kevin
The Oathbound (Mercedes Lackey, DAW, 1988) / Character: Tarma (magically induced)
The Bone People (Keri Hulme, Spiral Press, 1984) / Character: Kerewin

Webcomics:

Supernormal Step (Michael Lee Lunsford) / Character: Fiona
Ignition Zero (Noel Arthur Heimpel) / Characters: Orson and Robbie
Shades of A (Tab Kimpton) / Character: Anwar
Girls with Slingshots (Danielle Corsetto) / Character: Erin
Rain (Jocelyn Samara DiDomenick) / Characters: Chanel and Arthur

There are some celebrities who have come out as asexual, suggested themselves to be asexual at some time, or have claimed to be celibate due to lack of interest—a short list includes comedians Janeane Garofalo, Paula Poundstone, and Ben Rosen; writers J. M. Barrie, Keri Hulme, and Kenji Miyazawa; artist Edward Gorey; musicians Bradford Cox and Steven Morrissey; and fashion designers Tim Gunn and Karl Lagerfeld. (Note that some may have changed how they describe their orientation or don't mean "asexual" in the sense discussed in this book.)

Representation matters a *lot* to asexual people because there is so little of it. Most portrayals of people who do not have sex or are not interested in sex in media also include aberrant or non-human behavior; uninterested people are serial killers, aliens, mythical creatures, robots, or deeply damaged people who either have their lack of sexual interest used by the writers to show how strange or inhuman they are *or* are later "saved" or "made whole" by human emotion (in the form of a romantic relationship and sex). But when celebrities or mainstream media characters proudly or nonchalantly embrace an asexual identity (or, better yet, actually use the word *asexual* in a non-problematic way), asexual communities get very excited.

Unfortunately, asexual people are still the butt of jokes or presented as a big lie most of the time. A popular television show—the medical drama *House, M.D.*—featured an asexual-identified married couple as patients in a subplot of one episode.[44] It was a poor example, since the "asexual" man was debunked as suffering from a pituitary tumor inhibiting his sex drive and the "asexual" woman was found to be lying about her orientation to avoid making her husband feel guilty. The hero doctor of the episode, having debunked not one but two asexual people, concluded that "anyone who doesn't want sex is dead, dying, or lying," and the episode ended with asexuality "solved" as a sickness or a ruse. Asexual people reported having previously supportive friends and family see the episode and suddenly express concern for them, urging them to seek medical treatment.

And yet, that episode spurred a spike of interest in the topic. The Wikipedia article "Asexuality"[45] typically had around four thousand hits per day before the episode aired. The day it aired, more than fifty thousand people clicked through to the Wikipedia article, and the *Asexual Visibility and Education Network* beat its previous record for the most users online at once (most of whom were not registered). Many of these were probably people who had wondered whether they or someone they know might be asexual. If a show as mainstream as *House, M.D.* featured asexuality in a *positive* light, whether in a one-off or with a recurring asexual character, asexual people would be much better off.

<u>Asexual Community Insiders</u>

Not everyone who's asexual relates to the communities' beloved television shows or popular symbols (and some may even feel alienated by how enthusiastically other asexual people participate), but any group of people that shares space and intersects tends to develop a culture of sorts. Plenty of asexual people don't

---

44 "Better Half," *House, M.D.*, aired January 23, 2012.
45 en.wikipedia.org/wiki/Asexuality (Asexuality, 2002)

associate themselves with any of the following symbols or jokes, but here are a few themes that may pop up in asexual spaces.

Asexual people have a few inside jokes. They don't enjoy being mocked, but some are fond of poking fun at themselves, and one of the jokes sometimes thrown around is asexual people referring to themselves as *amoebas*. This refers to "asexual" being a type of reproduction when used in a biological context; sometimes, detractors suggest asexual people must be claiming to be plants or single-celled creatures if they use the word *asexual*. Reclaiming the taunt and using it in an empowering fashion, some asexual people enjoy the absurdity, but this and other dehumanizing terms have been used by outsiders to harass asexual people too, so non-asexual people should check for understanding before using it.

Especially on *AVEN*—the *Asexual Visibility and Education Network*—it is common to reference sharing and eating cake. This developed when some members discussed "what's better than sex?" and cake was the most popular answer. Cake is frequently featured in asexuality-related banners, logos, and blog names.

Asexual people have their own terms. Just like most heterosexual, homosexual, bisexual, polysexual, and pansexual people have shorthand ways of referring to their orientation (like straight, gay, bi, poly, and pan), asexual folks sometimes prefer to use a shorthand. Since just *a* sounds ridiculous and would be misunderstood easily, the term *ase* or *ace* developed (*ace* being far more popular because of how intuitive the spelling is), 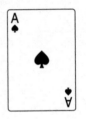 and from this, certain playing-card-related imagery cropped up (with Aces of Hearts sometimes used as symbols of romantic asexuality, and Aces of Spades assigned to aromanticism). As for graysexual and demisexual people, it's common to see *gray* and *grace*, and of course *demi*, or *demigrace/demigray* to cover both categories.

Some people, when referring to something or someone being appealing to asexual people or appealing in an asexual way, might call that thing or person *asexy*. It's sort of a joke, and sometimes also refers to something or someone being "sexy" with an acknowledgment that the asexual person saying so isn't actually expressing sexual attraction.

Asexual people who have romantic partners sometimes use traditional words to refer to them—words like *husband, wife, partner, significant other, boyfriend,* and *girlfriend*—but sometimes aromantic people use different words to describe their attraction to their partners. Some people will refer to the aromantic version of a crush as a *squish*. And some aromantic people with a queerplatonic partner might refer to their partner as their *zucchini*. (It's more or less an inside term that started as a joke to be a little absurd on purpose, but some people really do use it, and it's understood in many aromantic circles.)

A common scale used in describing sexual attraction is the Kinsey Scale. It allows people to describe their sexual orientation along a continuum, with "totally heterosexual" being a 0 on the scale and "totally homosexual" being a 6. The Kinsey Scale, while it has flaws, is relevant to asexual people because a value known as X was also included off the scale completely. It stood for people who don't feel any sexual attraction. Because of this, there are sometimes references to "being an X" or "on a scale of 0 to 6, I'm an X."

THE KINSEY SCALE (HETEROSEXUAL-HOMOSEXUAL RATING SCALE)[46]	
Rating	Description
0	Exclusively heterosexual
1	Predominantly heterosexual, only incidentally homosexual
2	Predominantly heterosexual, but more than incidentally homosexual
3	Equally heterosexual and homosexual
4	Predominantly homosexual, but more than incidentally heterosexual
5	Predominantly homosexual, only incidentally heterosexual
6	Exclusively homosexual
X	Non-sexual

Asexuality has its own flag. The flag was voted on by members of several separate asexual groups; there is no "president of asexuality," of course, and some people in the various communities don't like the flag and don't use it to represent themselves, but it's widely accepted. The flag is rectangular and  is made of four horizontal stripes of identical width. A black stripe on top stands for asexuality, a gray stripe underneath it stands for the gray areas (demisexuality, graysexuality), a white stripe underneath that represents asexuality allies, and the final stripe on the bottom is purple, symbolic of community.

Some asexual people have adopted an outward signal of their sexual orientation by wearing a black ring on their right middle finger. This is not widespread, and it's certainly not very likely to work as a recognizable signal to either other asexual people or sexually interested people who are considering propositions,

---

46 (Kinsey, 1948)

but some people like it as a regular reminder and some just think it's fun, and it's not uncommon to see black rings on the fingers of people who are participating in asexual awareness activities.

Asexuality has an awareness week. It has historically been celebrated in mid-October, but does not have firm dates as of this writing. The organization Asexual Awareness Week (www.asexualawarenessweek.com) is the best place to check for dates and events. Many asexual people celebrate Asexual Awareness Week by wearing asexual-friendly messages on their clothing, writing and sharing awareness materials, and even attending or organizing events. Colleges and universities often have gay/straight alliance organizations or LGBTQ clubs that include asexual people, and they sometimes plan panels with asexual guests or present an event like a documentary screening or awareness presentation. Mainstream press sometimes picks up stories for Asexual Awareness Week, and common understanding of asexual people is growing all the time.

Because asexual people frequently see a big difference between romantic attraction and sexual attraction (while most non-asexual people experience those elements as going hand in hand), asexual people often use complicated strings of terminology for something that seems like it should be simpler. It's not uncommon to encounter people describing themselves as "demisexual homoromantic" or "asexual demiromantic in a poly queerplatonic relationship," and wonder why they've analyzed themselves and their relationships to this degree.

But asexual people don't experience one or more of the aspects of traditional sexual and romantic attractions, and to figure out how their relationships can still work, they may have to unravel all the pieces and keep the ones that apply to them. Doing so often requires very specific terminology that may look overwhelming or even ridiculous at first glance. Rest assured they're not picking their feelings apart so exhaustively they don't have time to feel them properly (nor are they doing it as an attempt to confuse others). They just have to develop alternate models to figure out how they experience some but not all of the elements of intimacy and attraction, and they may need these tools to figure them out. Most other types of relationships have scripts and shorthand that everyone understands without explaining what attractions and experiences others can assume they entail; most asexual and especially aromantic relationships do not have these shortcuts.

As of this writing, popular places for asexual people to hang out online are *AVEN* (the *Asexual Visibility and Education Network*—lots of articles and forums);

LiveJournal's asexuality community (themed discussions with functional commenting, in blog format); Tumblr's various asexuality-themed blogs (largely image-heavy, with easy tracking of who and how many people are sharing and who's saying what); and various asexuality-themed groups on Facebook. These are discussed in more detail in the references section.

Non-Asexual People

In referring to people who do experience sexual attraction, some asexual people say "sexuals" or "sexual people," but a controversy erupted over this term because people who experience sexual attraction sometimes feel like it pigeonholes them or shames them (among other problems), representing them as being *defined* by the fact that they like sex or feel sexual attraction. And many people (especially people of color who are commonly sexualized no matter what they actually do) find it offensive or even triggering to be called "sexual." It's difficult to talk about the majority without naming it, but there seems to be some problem with just about every term that's been tried.

Non-asexual would exclude demisexual and graysexual people from discussions relevant to them. *Normatively sexual* excludes any sex outside of sex between two heterosexual cisgender partners. *Normal people* suggests anyone who is otherwise is *abnormal*, which is problematic. And *people who experience sexual attraction* is clunky.

Other attempts to establish a name for the majority include *allosexual* (prefix *allo-* means "other"), *consexual, monosexual, alisexual, *sexual*, and even *zedsexual* (like a reference to the opposite end of the alphabet from *asexual*), but none of these are universally accepted as of this writing. (*Allosexual* is probably in the widest use, but because it is easy to misinterpret its meaning as "people who are attracted to *all*," the term may fall out of usage.) Until or unless there's a term like *cisgender* (which developed when trans people wanted to refer to people who were not trans), disagreements will probably continue over this.

The Asexual Experience

Asexual people have a lot in common with each other even though they're also a diverse and varied group. Sometimes the diversity of the asexual population can make it difficult for a newly identified asexual person to figure out whether they fit in and whether they relate. If you are asexual or think you might be, Part Four of this book will help you with some of your questions, learning whether this label fits you, and figuring out how to navigate as an asexual person in a sexual world. And if you are a non-asexual person interested in understanding more about the asexual people in your life, Part Five is a great place to start.

PART THREE:
THE MANY MYTHS OF ASEXUALITY

Bingo!

A popular technique for collecting the common criticisms of any movement, identity, or experience is the "bingo card." Misunderstood groups use them to show how often they hear the same arguments, with every item on the card representing a misunderstanding or an inappropriate comment. Here's one example of an Asexuality Bingo Card:

B	I	N	G	O
That's a real shame because you're hot.	You must have been sexually abused as a child.	It's great that you're saving yourself.	You haven't met the right person.	You can't know you're asexual if you're a virgin.
If you tried it and didn't like it, you just did it wrong.	If you're sexually repulsed, you need therapy.	You're secretly gay.	Asexuality is an excuse for ugly people.	You can't be asexual if you masturbate.
You must have just gotten out of a bad relationship.	It's a phase. You'll grow out of it.	Get your hormones checked.	If it's really love, you'll want sex.	But humans are here to procreate!
The word for that is *abstinence*.	You'd be into sex if a hot celebrity propositioned you.	You must be a sociopath. Or a giant nerd.	You're just shy or scared. This is an excuse.	I could fix you—give me a chance!
You probably just never had an orgasm.	Everyone needs sex. You're repressing your desires.	You have no idea what you're missing.	So you think you're more "pure" than everyone else?	There's a pill for that.

Aren't They Using the Word *Asexual* Incorrectly?

"But that means you can reproduce by yourself!"

People who understand asexuality are often surprised to hear that asexual people *actually get this comment.* Yes, people make jokes about asexual people being "amoebas" or "plants" and turn it into an excuse to mock asexual people about how absurd asexuality is. What a silly group asexual people must be, using a term that means they can reproduce by budding!

Asexual people are not describing their *reproduction* with the term *asexual*. They're describing their *orientation*. And yet, detractors frequently pipe up with "I'm sorry, but I can't even consider your point of view because you're ruining a word that already has a meaning in *science.* That word is reserved for asexual *reproduction* and you're confusing people by expecting us to accept it!"

But language is always dependent on context. Scientific disciplines use context-dependent terms all the time. For instance, in a scientific context, *theory* has a totally different meaning from *theory* as used in a murder mystery or to describe a hunch. It would make no sense to say no one except scientists describing scientific theories can use the word *theory*. Similarly, asexuality can apply to someone's orientation. This word is not likely to confuse anyone. People claiming to be asexual are not actually making anyone legitimately wonder whether they are going to spontaneously clone themselves.

"But why don't they just say *abstinent* or *celibate*?" some people ask. It's true that many asexual people *do* practice abstinence because many of them aren't interested in having sex, but abstaining from sex is a practice, while asexuality is an orientation. Just like a gay man can have sex with a woman and still be gay, an asexual person can have sex and still not be sexually attracted to anyone, even the person with whom they share it. A percentage of asexual people are sexually active or have been in the past.

Anyone, regardless of sexual orientation, can choose to be abstinent. Nevertheless, despite the clear distinction between orientation and behavior, some people who don't want to acknowledge asexuality will still invoke "you're using the word wrong!" to avoid the issue. **If people are confused by asexuality, it's unlikely that it's because of the word.**

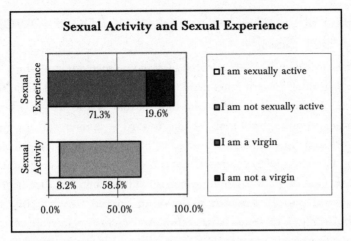

Sexual Activity and Sexual Experience

Sexual Experience — 71.3% — 19.6%

Sexual Activity — 8.2% — 58.5%

0.0%   50.0%   100.0%

☐ I am sexually active

▣ I am not sexually active

▣ I am a virgin

▪ I am not a virgin

Survey of self-identified asexual-spectrum people collected on the Internet September–October 2011[1]
Note: Because the survey was conducted on the Internet, the participating population skewed young. Older asexual people typically have more sexual experience.

Context has always been essential for determining meaning. For instance, *red* can apply to a color, a type of meat, a type of wine, a color of hair that's not actually the same as the crayon, an algal bloom causing discoloration in water, or the political alignment of a US state. But nobody tells redheads to stop calling themselves *redheads* because that word is reserved for conversations about alcoholic beverages, and no one tells the political commentators not to use *red state* because of possible confusion about red tides or steak. Nobody flails and protests these uses as "confusing," because the context makes it 100 percent clear.

You don't assume someone described as "hot" must need a cold drink. You don't assume someone is sitting on punctuation if they say they're on their period. You don't *actually* think an asexual person is going to reproduce through asexual reproduction, so the argument that it is confusing is absolutely ridiculous.

Asexual is also sometimes accused of being a made-up sexuality, a "new" and therefore unofficial/inappropriate term, or a placeholder people use until they find their "real" sexuality. **Invalidation takes many forms, but the shallowest of them all manifests in denying asexual people access to language that describes them.** Mocking the word itself as a means of calling asexuality fake, pointless, or absurd is a fairly superficial method, but it does have the effect of silencing these conversations by making them seem ridiculous or petty. Asexual people should be the authorities on what terms they use to describe themselves, and allies of asexual people should learn their language instead of expecting to control it.

---

1 Community Census. (Asexual Awareness Week, 2011)

Is Asexuality Based on Fear of or Anger Toward Other Genders?

Sometimes asexual people are accused of avoiding sexual relationships because of negative feelings toward other genders. (LGBTQ people deal with this accusation too.) As they fail to understand that asexual people are describing their attraction experiences—not their feelings toward or opinions of any gender— these critics sometimes insist the cause of a person's asexuality is a gender-based hatred or a previous bad experience that causes anxiety based on gender.

Just like a lesbian's attraction to women is not by definition a statement against men, **asexual people are not expressing hatred toward any gender through their lack of sexual attraction**. And just like gay men are not attracted to men as a fear reaction toward women, asexual people aren't defined by fear and avoidance of intimacy to the point that attraction can't develop. If a person who is asexual does happen to express negative feelings toward any gender and has a pattern of doing so, there may be something psychological or pathological going on, but this should never be assumed, especially in the absence of any evidence, and any hate being expressed is not automatically the cause of a person's lack of attraction.

Some asexual people do get upset with those who routinely proposition them for sex, try to talk them out of being asexual, tell them they're going to waste by not having sex, or make sexually charged statements to provoke them. Because asexual people who receive this treatment do not always respond calmly to these comments, their anger with particular members of whatever gender pursues them can sometimes be misinterpreted as hatred for the entire gender, and in rare cases, if the harassment is egregious enough, it may actually cause misdirected hate or distrust. It *can* happen, even though it usually doesn't, but when it does, it shouldn't be assumed to be the cause of asexuality. It's much more likely to be a side effect of unwanted attention.

There is also the related suggestion that asexual people—especially asexual women— are actually *demonstrating* hatred of whatever gender is propositioning them through the very act of refusing to

> I'm not saying that I stayed in bad relationships because I didn't know I was asexual and aromantic. But I am saying that if I had realized, had known what those things were, had realized that asexuality and not sexism explained my experiences—I might have made different decisions."
> —AYDAN SELBY, *THE ASEXUAL AGENDA*

sleep with them. This is patently ridiculous and sexist. **Not being attracted to someone—and therefore not engaging in sexual activity with**

that person—doesn't constitute hateful treatment. It also doesn't demonstrate fear. Sometimes asexual people are told they should be indifferent to sex, and therefore should just shrug and go through with it if someone wants them to. It's very wrong to tell any person, asexual or not, what sexual experiences they are obligated to consent to.

Asexual people aren't automatically demonstrating fear of the potential sex partner—or of sex itself—if they say they're not willing to engage in it. Some people may fear sexual experiences or specific people who desire them sexually, but even when that's the case, it cannot be successfully addressed through harassment, repeated propositions, or cajoling the person into sex expecting to change their orientation. It is frankly no one's business if any person's attitude toward sex includes fear; avoiding experiences perceived as unpleasant or scary is not unreasonable, and those who repeatedly try to pressure asexual people into "getting over" what they perceive as fear are not providing the eye-opening tough love they think they are. No one should decide—supposedly for the asexual person's own good—that sexual experiences need to be imposed on another person.

There's a popular perception that people who aren't sexually active need help to become so (and that they will thank their "coaches" afterward), but these kinds of experiences need to be controlled by the individual. People who are reluctant to engage in sexual relationships for any reason are unlikely to be grateful to someone who keeps trying to change them and refuses to listen. It's more likely a person who is persistent about imposing sexual experiences on another will only be treated with mistrust and estrangement.

Do People Become Asexual Because They Fail at Dating?

Predictably, the answer is no. Asexual people are actually very likely to have dated in the past, to be actively dating, or to be in relationships (if they're so inclined). Most asexual people get the same amount of romantic attention that anyone else

> "Here was a friendly, attractive woman who obviously wanted me. No one had ever expressed an interest in me like this before. She wanted to do this for months. I wanted nothing. And I just sat there. *This isn't right.* Why didn't I want her? Why didn't I feel anything? Why couldn't I feel anything? What is wrong with me?"
> —TOM, *ASEXUALITY ARCHIVE*

with similar characteristics would get, unless they feel compelled to avoid contact with others out of fear that unwanted propositions will come up. (Most asexual people do not avoid having social lives, incidentally.) Sometimes they're very perplexed by the romantic/sexual attention they do get because they may not feel comfortable responding to it or don't quite understand why sexual attention always seems to be an expected part of romance, but none of this means they must be dating failures.

"You just can't get anyone" is a very common suggestion by people who want to dismiss asexuality. This is inspired by failure to empathize. Most people want sexual relationships; therefore, if they think about how *they* would feel without sexual attraction or sexual relationships, some imagine the asexual person must feel desperation and despair. These types of people may not understand the concept of "single" without considering it synonymous with "looking" or may not understand being happy without sexual experiences. They may not understand what it means to not yearn to be part of a couple or partnership. That's why they can't look at an asexual person (especially a person who does not want to date) and process the idea of that person being happy. Asexuality becomes, in their minds, much more understandable as a convenient explanation chosen by a person who's embarrassed about finding no suitable partners.

Asexuality is not a synonym for "people who have experienced resounding rejection their whole lives." Furthermore, people don't "become asexual." **Bad experiences do not make people stop being sexually attracted to others, nor does "giving up" on finding a partner.** There are plenty of people who do indeed get frustrated over dating-related difficulties, and asexual people who date are not exempt from this, but someone who has given up on dating is not the same as someone who is asexual.

Being an introvert, being shy, being socially awkward, being undesirable in some way, having low self-esteem, and being angry at the world are all descriptions frequently thrown at asexual people to invalidate them, too, and all of these fail to "explain" asexuality for the same reasons as those discussed above. An asexual person—like any other person—might have some of these qualities, but when someone is heterosexual and has these qualities, we don't say they are definitive of heterosexuality. The same is true of asexuality. Allies of asexual people will not point to aspects of their personality that might complicate all sorts of social relationships and blame these traits for their orientation.

Do People Become Asexual Because They're Physically Unattractive?

Again, no. People don't stop having sexual attraction to others because they themselves are not conventionally attractive. Asexual people's sexual orientation is not dependent on availability of partners; it is dependent on their own inclinations.

Other people's opinions of someone's looks don't dictate their ability to feel attracted to others. "Being ugly" doesn't make sex drive or sexual attraction go away. Unfortunately, people who want to dismiss asexuality will often say "I wouldn't sleep with you anyway" to individual asexual people—a suggestion that their own aesthetic choice of who's suitable to sleep with is the ultimate test of whether someone is "too ugly." Attractiveness is extremely subjective, though, and people who drop judgments about who's too ugly to get sex tend to present these assessments as objective.

This kind of comment also targets fat people who identify as asexual. Even though plenty of heavy people find partners, *fat* is often weaponized as a synonym for *undesirable* and/or *ugly*. People who are overweight are frequently desexualized no matter what their orientation and are subjected to damaging comments and attitudes regarding their eligibility as dating and sex partners. Asexual people who are also fat are often assumed to be identifying as such due to lack of willing partners or as a natural physical consequence of being unhealthy and are expected to start desiring or pursuing sex only if they lose weight. **Of course, being fat is not synonymous with being unhealthy, and it is also not synonymous with having no available partners or with having no sex drive or inclination.** The assumption that fat asexual people are identifying as asexual *because* they're fat is disappointingly common.

That said, there is no known correlation between being asexual and being physically unattractive. Asexual people may be less inclined to conform to aesthetic expectations in some cases, but they are not, as a general rule, less aesthetically attractive people. Like most populations, asexual people run the gamut of attractiveness; there will surely be a few very unattractive people in the pool, as well as a few gorgeous people. Most people are somewhere in between. If the attractiveness spectrum didn't include at least some people who are less normatively attractive, it wouldn't be a normal distribution.

Non-asexual people who possess below-average attractiveness aren't excluded as a group from all opportunities for sex and relationships. It's not as if all "ugly" non-asexual people never find mates or get married. The standards of who is eligible for mating are not entirely dependent on physical appearance. Anyone of any orientation can become frustrated with lack of willing partners, but asexual people haven't become asexual because of their appearance (regardless of what it is). Many asexual people describe feeling annoyed or harassed or bewildered by romantic and sexual attention; it isn't as though getting offers changes their orientation.

Desire for positive sexual attention is not the only reason a person might want to be attractive. Sometimes asexual people hear "why would you dress like that/do your hair that way/wear makeup if you aren't trying to attract a partner?" This is, of course, a misleading question because grooming oneself isn't a universally deliberate signal for sex or romantic attention no matter who it comes from. Partnered people do not (usually) completely stop wearing attractive clothing or doing their beauty/grooming routines once they get a partner, and the continued attempts to look good are not exclusively for the benefit of the partner(s). Many people report that looking good makes them feel good, which doesn't necessarily imply any relationship with wanting to appear attractive in a sexual context. It should never be assumed that a person who is attractive or is perceived to have done something to be more aesthetically pleasing is therefore trying to get a partner (or is a tease).

Asexual people can often care about their looks just as much as anyone else and can sometimes suffer from body image issues and dysmorphia, eating disorders, low self-esteem related to their looks, and mental illnesses tied in with their physical presentation. They are not living in a bubble away from the judgment of society just because most of them are not deliberately hoping their bodies will be attractive enough to help them get sexual partners.

In short, asexual people's physical appearance—regardless of whether it attracts partners—is not an attribute anyone should use to invalidate their orientation.

Do Asexual People Have a Physical or Hormonal Problem?

Asexuality is not thought to be linked to any biological disease or disorder (no matter what they said on *House, M.D.*). Most asexual people have typical bodies, bodily functions,[2] and hormone production. Asexual people are just as likely as non-asexual people to become aroused if stimulated.[3] Some describe a lower-than-average sex drive or lack of arousal experiences, but the strength of someone's sex drive is not the key determining factor of their orientation.

Monitoring one's health is certainly a good idea. If an asexual person or a family member/friend of an asexual person is concerned that the asexual person may have an illness, they can be checked for a few disorders that cause a decline in sexual interest (though, again, sexual interest is not sexual attraction).

---

2 When both asexual and non-asexual people had their functions measured while watching a film: "There were no significant group differences in the increased VPA and self-reported sexual arousal response to the erotic film between the groups." (Brotto & Yule, "Physiological and Subjective Sexual Arousal in Self-Identified Asexual Women," 2011)

3 "[T]he findings suggest normal subjective and physiological sexual arousal capacity in asexual women and challenge the view that asexuality should be characterized as a sexual dysfunction." (Brotto & Yule, "Physiological and Subjective Sexual Arousal in Self-Identified Asexual Women," 2011)

There are hormone disorders[4] and sexual arousal/genital-related disorders that interact with ability to have or enjoy or want sex,[5] and psychological conditions exist. A person can suffer from erotophobia (irrational fear of sex or something related to it), genophobia (fear of sexual intercourse), sexual anorexia (pathological loss of sexual appetite and/or fear of romance and intimacy), or anhedonia (the inability to experience pleasure, including sexual pleasure). They can experience sexual interest/arousal disorder (lack of interest or reduced interest) or hypoactive sexual desire disorder. **However, lack of sexual interest or attraction is not the only symptom in any of these disorders.**

Biology isn't always irrelevant to sexual orientation; for instance, some intersex individuals identify as asexual. Many intersex variations exist and some of them involve hormone production or sensitivity/immunity issues.[6] Some intersex people may not experience some aspects of puberty due to hormone irregularities, and because hormone disorders have other biological consequences, these folks may choose to have some form of hormone regimen or alternate therapy (if available). A person with an intersex variation can still be asexual without it being "an illness"; it's not helpful to blame the intersex person's biology to dismiss the orientation, even though everyone's biology interacts with their orientation and psychology.

People with disabilities also sometimes identify as asexual. As a group that faces desexualization fairly often, asexual people with disabilities are frequently told their attitude toward sex is just a result of internalized oppression, but yes, people can be asexual and have a disability.[7] An asexual person is not less asexual even if some aspects of their sex life, sexual attitude, or sexual interest might *interact* with some aspects of the rest of their lives, including their disabilities.

Some people who are on medication for physical or mental illnesses may experience a lower or absent sex drive because of the medication.[8] Especially when the condition requiring these medicines is chronic, these people sometimes develop no sexual interest in others and are sometimes comfortable identifying as asexual. When a medical condition or its treatment interferes with or interacts

---

4 An imbalance, absence, or sensitivity/immunity to various hormones—androgens (testosterone, androstenedione, dehydroepiandrosterone), estrogens (estradiol, estrone, estriol), progesterone, and prolactin—can affect sexual desire. (Regan, 1999)

5 "Sexual pain disorders include dyspareunia and vaginismus." (Phillips, 2000)

6 Various chromosomal, hormonal, and anatomy-related conditions exist under the intersex umbrella. isna.org includes a list. (Intersex Society of North America, 2008)

7 "While asexuality has been persistently criticized as a damaging myth imposed on disabled people, individuals with disabilities who do not identify as sexual highlight the inseparable intersection between normality and sexuality." (Kim, 2011)

8 "Many commonly used drugs can interfere with sexual function in both men and women, causing loss of libido, interfering with erection or ejaculation in men, and delaying or preventing orgasm in women." (Medical Letter on Drugs and Therapeutics, 1992)

with a person's appetite for sex, it's fine to acknowledge that it may be partially "responsible," or at least influential, without trying to tell these people they're "not really asexual." **Orientation is complicated, and a person does *not* have to be free of all possible complicating factors to be asexual.**

Before suggesting that the asexuality might be caused by physical or mental disorders, curious parties should ask themselves a) whether the asexual person's medical history is any of their business, and b) in cases where it *is* any of their business, whether any *other* physical symptoms or significant changes in the asexual person's attitude toward sexual attraction, sexual interest, or sexual experiences have cropped up. If the answer is no, it's more appropriate to acknowledge the possibility that this person is asexual rather than trying to find some medical problem that could be causing it. Assuming a disorder must be responsible is an ineffective and possibly offensive way to approach discussion about asexuality.

All this said, wanting to encourage another person's "optimal health" is often a misguided quest. Unless one is directly responsible for the health and safety of a person who cannot make their own decisions, other people's medical and lifestyle choices should be respectfully left to the individual. Pressuring them to change their habits, pursue possibly unnecessary tests and procedures (that may or may not be stressful, expensive, ineffective, or painful), or adopt alternate ideas about health is inappropriate.

Asexual is what people call themselves if they aren't sexually attracted to other people. It doesn't matter whether a little, some, most, or all of the reason that someone isn't sexually attracted to anyone has to do with some other aspect of their lives. There are many ways to be asexual. It's a label asexual people put on themselves to describe what they're experiencing, not why they're experiencing it.

Are Asexual People Too Distracted by Their Busy Lives to Be Sexual?

Sometimes detractors have a misconception regarding asexual people being too preoccupied with other aspects of their lives to "properly" pursue sexual relationships. There's a popular conception of asexual people "throwing themselves into" some other passion to distract themselves from failures that would inevitably result if they tried to pursue romantic/sexual interests. Again, this is just a result of people projecting their own coping strategies onto others. It's not an explanation for asexuality.

People chase their passions. If a partner-desiring asexual person has an interest in someone, they dedicate the necessary time to cultivating that relationship in whatever way they wish. As for non-partner-desiring asexual people, sure some may spend more time alone and may fill that time with solitary pursuits, but many of them have active social lives and close non-romantic/non-partner relationships

> "We shouldn't feel pressured to provide reasons in a quest to convince others that our choices are valid. It can be hard to own a status that some people may consider embarrassing, but then again, it will always be embarrassing unless people own up. Whether we were 'too busy' or 'career focused' or 'waiting for the one,' we just did not feel like having sex."
> —ILY, *ASEXY BEAST*

that require time and energy. It's not a case of being unable to dig out room in a packed schedule for this one type of relationship that's supposed to trump all others.

When something matters to a person, they invest time and energy into pursuing it. It makes no sense to suggest that, in the case of asexual people, they must have just put a cap on what their lives can contain and left out the part that involves sex or relationships. If someone feels a desire for it, that person can, of course, choose to ignore it if a career or a project is determined to be more important, but ignoring urges or crushes is not what asexuality is. **If people are asexual, it's not because they ran out of time to have sexual relationships.**

Funnily enough, asexual people are also sometimes "accused" of having *too much* free time—and asked why they haven't won a Nobel Prize or cured cancer since they surely must be doing something immensely constructive with all that time not spent on pursuing sex. The "but what do you *do* all day??" response is not uncommon, but this is more insulting to non-asexual people than to asexual people, considering it implies that non-asexual orientations prevent one from being productive or dominate one's attention entirely. Most of the vastly productive people in the world are not asexual. And being asexual does not guarantee that one will have abundant free time.

Since most people do perceive sexual and/or romantic relationships as central to life, it's not surprising that they see those who don't desire those relationships as having "extra" free time. Yes, someone may have more free time if they're not engaging in a time-consuming activity that nearly everyone else feels compelled to pursue. But that's like suggesting a person who pursued basketball as a career did so "instead of" pursuing a career in baseball. Most non-partner-seeking people don't feel their activities are "instead of" partner seeking.

Viewing partnered and/or sexually active life as the default, and all other arrangements as deviations, is not an accurate, useful, or supportive perspective for an asexual ally to maintain.

Did Asexual People Have a Bad Sexual Experience and Swear Off Sex?

This question demonstrates a "can't win" situation. If an asexual person is a virgin, they're taunted with "you can't know until you try it," but if the asexual person *has* had sex, some detractors are convinced that it must have been unpleasant, carried out improperly, or experienced "with the wrong person," forever soiling their opinion of sex. **Blaming the sex an asexual person has had is very common, and it's unfortunate because bad sex doesn't cause people to stop experiencing sexual attraction.** (Of course, if someone never has anything but bad sex experiences, that person might get soured on sex eventually, but it doesn't mean the person stops being attracted to others.)

Some asexual people who have decided they want to try sex despite not feeling sexually attracted to anyone *do*, in fact, have bad sex experiences, or at least go through with it and really find it difficult to see what the fuss is about. (One doesn't have to be asexual to have this reaction, of course.) Being sexually attracted to one's partner(s)—including the lead-up of wanting it and having that urge satisfied—often greatly enhances the experience of sex, and if an asexual person doesn't have that dimension, the actual sex part may be anywhere from physically enjoyable to actively gross and/or unpleasant. **Scratching usually feels a lot better if you've already got an itch.**

Sexual Experience of Self-Identified Asexual-Spectrum People

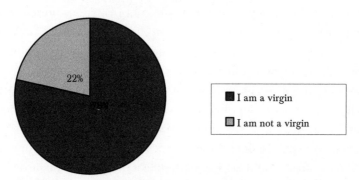

22%

■ I am a virgin

■ I am not a virgin

Reported in one survey of self-identified asexual-spectrum people collected on the Internet September–October 2011.[9] The surveyed population skews young because it was administered through Internet communities, and of the 3,436 respondents, less than 20 percent were older than age 25, with 76 percent being between ages 16 and 24. Older asexual people typically have had more sexual experience.

---

9 Community Census. (Asexual Awareness Week, 2011)

Some asexual people do feel like they "need" to go through with a sexual act just to see if they can jump-start themselves; there are asexual people out there who worry that something is wrong with them and wonder whether everyone's right—that having sex may actually "cure" them. This is pretty common in asexual people who haven't heard of asexuality; they may search fruitlessly for a sexual situation they feel motivated toward, can enjoy, or can at least tolerate, and they can get frustrated and desperate when they don't feel what people say they're supposed to feel (while, of course, probably frustrating or confusing their partners who don't understand what they might be doing wrong and may blame themselves).

Sexual attraction and interest isn't like vampirism. It isn't passed on once a person is "bitten." Most non-asexual virgins are well aware that they want to have sex; they need no help. Feeling left out of what everyone else seems to desire can be very isolating, so it's common for asexual people to push their comfort zones in an attempt to be like everyone else.

It's not terribly uncommon for an asexual person to try sex and think it's pretty good or not bad. Some who aren't too put off by sex with a person they're not attracted to may enjoy the physical sensations and maybe the emotional intimacy, but the experience of sex does not change how

> "I've had sex. It wasn't a compromise. It wasn't solely for her pleasure. It wasn't to save the relationship. It wasn't a violation. I did it for me. I did it because I wanted to experience it. On the whole, it was positive. It felt good. I liked it. But ... it wasn't the mindblowing experience I was led to believe. It didn't sexually awaken me. I didn't start craving sex with every waking hour of my life. I didn't suddenly start to feel sexually attracted to her or anyone else. I felt like I was acting. That was nine years ago. I haven't had sex since. I don't miss it."
> —TOM, ASEXUALITY ARCHIVE

they experience attraction. However, most asexual people who try sex say they *didn't* enjoy it (and found it alienating that they didn't enjoy it) and certainly aren't encouraged by the experience to try to find a different partner or a different style of sex they can then try to like. After society tells asexual people for years that they'll love this and then they don't, they're often less likely to blithely continue experimenting while hoping the world will be right about the next one.

Many people who say bad sex is to blame for asexuality simply can't imagine not enjoying the experience. These people might gain some semblance of understanding if they tried to imagine having sex with a person who was in no way physically attractive to them—someone who was the wrong gender for their preference, or the wrong body type, or in the wrong age range. If a person who has trouble believing sex could be unenjoyable can imagine a person they are not attracted to *at all*, and then try to imagine whether they could enjoy sex with that person, they might have some understanding of how an asexual person *might* be feeling about sex. Many asexual people feel that way about *all* potential partners. Just like most straight guys can't imagine liking sex with another man, many asexual people would not enjoy the act—not because they're doing it wrong, but because people just aren't sexually attractive to them.

So, for asexual people, regardless of whether they've had bad sex, asexuality is likely to be the *cause* of their attitude toward those experiences, not the result. If a straight guy had sex with a man and told people he'd hated it because he didn't think he was gay, most people wouldn't say "no, you must've just had bad gay sex, keep trying" or "no, you must've just had gay sex with the wrong partner, try someone else." They'd usually believe him. Asexual people should be treated no differently.

Could Asexual People Be Suffering From Trauma Brought on by Sexual Abuse?

Unfortunately, sexual abuse and other types of abuse are a reality in this world. Some people who experience sexual abuse or sexual harassment become sex-averse, at least for a time.[10] And since experiencing sexual attraction is considered normal, some folks dream up a cause for asexual people's disinterest instead of processing what asexual people say. Assign trauma to the people they don't understand, and presto!—they don't have to reexamine their assumptions about how "everyone" actually wants sex.

You must have been abused is a phrase asexual people hear all the time. First, a message to anyone who might consider saying this: ***do not bring up abuse without warning in any conversation.*** Some people who unthinkingly toss out this comment as a dismissal don't realize that, if it is actually true, it's an incredibly insensitive thing to say. If someone thinks an asexual person was so emotionally scarred by an assault or abuse experience that it changed their sexual orientation, it definitely should not be brought up unexpectedly. A person's possible trigger reactions shouldn't be considered less important than a skeptic's desire to squash the so-called asexual person's identity by writing it off as psychological trauma. This is not something to joke about or invoke dismissively.

---

10 "[S]exual aversion disorder has many, often interrelated, causes. Incest, molestation, rape and psychological abuse are often factors resulting in a woman developing complete avoidance of physical intimacy and revulsion at the thought of sexual touch." (Banner, Whipple & Graziottin, 2006)

But what if the critic doesn't mean it that way and doesn't actually think the asexual person was abused?

. . . Well, then why is it suggested in the first place? And how could anyone be sure of what the person they're speaking to has experienced?

Some people make this comment because they want to use very strong words to silence another person. The argument often follows this pattern: "You're not asexual; you were obviously abused. If you don't remember it, it must have happened before your memory kicks in." This is obviously a no-win situation—and a bad argument, since the person who makes it has already decided asexuality makes sense only if the person was traumatized by abuse; therefore, it *must have happened.* This is a very weak technique to undermine asexuality, at the expense of another person, argued by someone who either does not realize or does not care about the damage it might cause. **No one should suggest abuse is at the root of someone else's sexual orientation.**

It does make sense that people *wonder* about abuse or trauma. If you are a non-asexual person who wants to ask this question of an asexual person you're talking to, the best thing to do is avoid the topic unless you are explicitly invited down that road. If the asexual person opens up about abuse—either to say it happened or that it didn't—you might try asking if you can ask a personal question about their experience. There are some asexual people who are open about this, but if they don't bring it up, you shouldn't push the conversation in that direction. This information is best discussed between the (possibly) affected person, that person's loved ones/family/trusted friends, and if applicable, that person's therapist/mental health professional(s). But since people are curious about how asexual people may be affected by abuse, it will be discussed here.

Not being attracted to anyone or being disinclined to pursue sex is not a sign of something deeply scarring in a person's past. Just like some people still spread the message that men turn gay because they were molested as boys, or that gay women are only lesbians because a man hurt them or disappointed them, there are those who believe everyone is sexually attracted to others as a default and anything that leads to a different orientation should be fixed. These folks believe mental trauma could be blocking a person's ability to feel attraction.

Let's first acknowledge that abuse does happen (unfortunately). A subset of the asexual population has been abused (sexually or otherwise). That's because a subset of any population experiences abuse. In cases of asexual people who were abused before maturity, it will of course be difficult to tease out how much

> "I hate this question because it falls into a tendency to search for causation that belies a need to pathologize. No one ever asks heterosexual individuals what caused their sexual orientation. When we ask individuals what 'causes' some part of them, we are saying, 'Do you know why this thing is wrong with you?' We are also saying, 'If you do know, do you think we could change it so this doesn't happen to anyone else?'"
>
> —M. LeClerc, *Hypomnemata*

the abuse influenced the lens through which they see the world. In cases of asexual people who were maturing or mature before the traumatic event(s) or abusive living situation(s), they will have often been aware of their asexual tendencies before the abuse.

And, unfortunately, there have been cases of asexual people experiencing "corrective" rape. This is when a person gets assaulted *for* being asexual; the attacker believes the asexual person will learn that sex is fun and "reconsider" being asexual if forced to engage in it. This, sadly, is perpetrated in a "corrective" fashion by people who know the victim and may even be in a relationship with them. Because of society's common sex-compulsory narrative, asexual victims can sometimes be made to feel as though their attackers and abusers had the right to demand sex, or may at least feel unworthy of relationships if they do not have sex. Using abuse and sexual assault in an attempt to make an asexual person accept sex is a violent act, not a wake-up call.

No matter how an abuse experience has affected an asexual person's willingness to have sex, their view of sexual subjects, or their attraction experiences in general, it is not appropriate to say that their asexuality is inauthentic because of it. Nobody else gets to decide that what another person has been through negates their self-concept.

Keep in mind that most people who have had an unpleasant, unwanted sexual experience still continue to experience sexual attraction.[11] Sexual abuse can be a horrible, scarring experience, but it generally does not forever remove the victim's ability to see others as sexually attractive. It is good to seek counseling if sexual abuse has caused lasting trauma, but it should never be with the intent of declaring asexuality a symptom. Aversion to sex as a trauma reaction manifests as fear and disgust, not lack of attraction.

There are also asexual people who were (and are) affected by neglect, violence, or emotional abuse, and they are sometimes condescendingly told their

---

11 "Social and sexual functioning are substantially disrupted immediately following the rape and tend to return to pre-rape levels after a few months, although sexual satisfaction remains low up to 18 months later." (Steketee & Foa, 1987)

asexuality is not a valid orientation, but is rather a natural function of having bad models or lacking models for healthy relationships. Asexual people who have these experiences may have trouble with intimacy—as anyone in that situation might—but it's still inaccurate to say a person who feels no sexual attraction or doesn't pursue sex is only oriented that way because they were never properly taught how to love, are modeling the distant behavior of their abusers, or are afraid of other people because of past violence.

It is always *possible* that a person could be hiding shame surrounding trauma behind the label of asexuality. People do sometimes misuse labels, whether intentionally, accidentally, or through ignorance. The point is that asexuality should never be suggested to probably or definitely be a symptom following from abuse. There are few contexts in which it is appropriate to discuss someone's personal abuse history and bringing it up to deny that their sexual identity is not one of those contexts.

Sometimes asexual people who have experienced abuse of some kind will want to seek counseling, and especially if that abuse was sexual, the counselor or mental health professional will often be predisposed to assuming lack of sexual attraction or interest is a trauma reaction. Asexual clients can have a much better therapy experience if they inquire about the therapist's friendliness toward asexuality first. A good starting point might be a therapist with a background in LGBT issues; they tend to be trained better in respecting non-heteronormative identities. They should be able to work with an asexual client who wants to address trauma without focusing on the client's ability to have or desire sexual relationships as a sign of success.

Therapy-seeking asexual people may consider a pre-session interview with their mental health professionals during which they can ascertain whether the therapist acknowledges asexuality as an orientation. They can point to the *Diagnostic and Statistical Manual of Mental Disorders*—the *DSM-5*—as a trusted resource that accepts asexuality as an exception to some diagnosable sex-related disorders, and they may choose to bring recently published scientific studies on the asexual population to show the mental health professional that others in the field are taking it seriously—and therefore, so should they.

Could Asexual People Be Secretly Gay?

Many asexual people ask themselves this question before they realize they're asexual. (And they may even continue to wonder whether they're just repressing homosexuality after identifying tentatively as asexual for some time.)

> "So, having realized that I wasn't becoming in-
> terested in guys in the way that was expected,
> the next logical conclusion was that maybe I
> was interested in girls instead? That was quickly
> disproved though—I tried looking at girls, and
> thinking about girls, etc. but it didn't do anything
> for me either."
> —MARY KAME GINOZA, *NEXT STEP: CAKE*

People are taught that they're expected to like cross-sex partners. When asexual people find themselves not feeling heterosexual attraction, they look at the orientations available to them and sometimes think being gay is the only other option. They may also think they are bisexual, polysexual, or pansexual. Observing that their interest in one gender is the same as any other, they may pick up one of the terms that seems to describe that, without realizing asexuality is a possibility.

When people ask whether asexual-identified people are actually gay and deliberately hiding it, they're suggesting that they must be so ashamed of being gay that they publicly claim an orientation in which chastity is expected.

One problem with "you're probably gay" is that asexuality is also a misunderstood, marginalized orientation. **If someone is gay and wanting to hide it, pretending to be asexual instead is not a good way to make life easier.** Asexual people have a different experience from gay people, but they are still badgered and questioned and disbelieved and disrespected and attacked and denied and tossed into obscurity. There might be a perception that asexual people do not have to deal with the same persecution that gay people do, and while that is often true (unless the asexual person in question is also LGB+), they get a different negative experience. Asexuality isn't a shortcut out of getting picked on for one's sexual orientation, and it is not necessarily "easier."

It is worth noting that prejudice against homosexuality in religious or very conservative families or environments might lead some closeted gay folks to believe coming out as asexual would be less frowned upon. And in some situations, they'd be right. However, most closeted gay people who worry about repercussions will pose as heterosexual, not asexual. Presenting asexuality as an orientation to an unsympathetic audience will result in a different reaction—though it's more likely to inspire confusion than the violent reaction one might expect when coming out as gay—but since asexuality isn't "I'm waiting until marriage to have sex," it will still be criticized and dismissed and considered unnatural by the same people if they actually understand what it is. It's being non-heterosexual, not being gay, that inspires unpleasant reactions.[12]

---

12 "[T]hose liking (or disliking) homosexuals or bisexuals likewise like (or dislike) asexuals." (MacInnis & Hodson, 2012)

Some members of LGBTQ communities protest that asexuality awareness might be dangerous to their community because LGBTQ people have been historically shamed into not having sex. They may believe asexuality awareness will help reinforce this persecution and oppression, since more awareness about the orientation may lead homophobes to "sell" asexuality as a choice. However, this is misleading, because homophobes are really trying to sell LGBTQ people a choice between heterosexuality or a life of abstinence, and no one who understands what asexuality is will claim it is a synonym for chastity. This issue is discussed in more detail in Part Two of this book.

"You're probably gay and too ashamed to admit it" is what people assume when they have not grown past seeing the world in tight dichotomies—so to them, a person claiming to be asexual should be put in the not-straight box, which is labeled "gay" in their minds.

Most asexual people who come out to disbelieving others are subjecting themselves to a humbling experience that has them feeling vulnerable; and not only that, but they're also committing to explaining what asexuality *is*. People know what homosexuality is, and while some gay people face violent or disapproving reactions if they come out, they do not get told that no one feels the way they feel, and they probably aren't going to have to explain what homosexuality is to nearly everyone they come out to.

Some claim that asexuality is an escape for those who want to avoid admitting their non-straight, queer, or kinky desires. That it's some kind of criticism-free, virtuous island that is respected and revered

> "It is not okay within mainstream society for a woman to never express sexual desire. It is certainly not okay to be openly, loudly asexual, and it is damn well not the ideal for women to be asexual. Where do you think the term *frigid* comes from? Did you think it was a compliment?"
>
> —SCIATRIX, *WRITING FROM FACTOR X*

because of its popular association with chastity. That it's the only way some closeted gay people can avoid the gay stigma without being expected to have straight sex. The truth is that **asexual people are expected to have straight sex too. They aren't respected or left alone.** Their personal lives are pried into as well. Their life choices are brought into the open and spread out by people demanding justification and proof. People are expected to be sexually active. Asexuality is not a way out. It doesn't work as an escape.

And, of course, when it comes to gay asexual people (as well as those in non-heteronormative relationships, or with said inclinations), this suggestion is even sillier. LGBTQ asexual people can get all the fun of being harassed for their LGBTQ identity or orientation, and then they can be harassed for their asexuality on top of that.

The bottom line is that people who say they are sexually attracted to no one mean exactly that. It's absurd how often asexual people say "I'm not attracted to anyone" and hear "so . . . you're gay then?" in response. Sexual orientation is not an either/or situation. You can't have a multiple-choice question regarding "Who are you attracted to?" and only offer "A. the same gender," "B. other genders," and "C. both" without acknowledging that there should be an option for "D. none." This also oversimplifies gender, of course. But the main point is that "asexual" is indeed "not heterosexual" while not being homosexual either.

This question is often motivated by the belief that *everyone* is attracted to *something*. This misconception usually manifests as "you're gay if you're not straight," but some detractors will take this even further and assign the asexual person a secret attraction to animals or inanimate objects. No, asexuality is not a cover for zoophilia or objectum sexuality. It is absurd to interpret a lack of heterosexuality as a blank that can be filled with any hypothetical attraction experience.

Have Asexual People Just Not Met the Right Person?

It's possible. Asexual people may have not met the right person to be sexually attracted to. It's possible in the same way that heterosexual people may not have met the right person of the same gender to make them realize they're not straight. It's possible in the same way that men who don't wear traditionally feminine clothes may not have found the right dress to make them comfortable with cross-dressing. It is possible in the same way that people who hate ground beef may have just not had the right hamburger.

In a very distantly possible, scientific sense, *yes*, of course it's possible that an asexual person who has never been sexually attracted to anyone *could* encounter someone in the world who inspires sexual attraction for them. If an experience is possible for most people, it makes sense to suggest that maybe a person who hasn't experienced it still might. But responding to a non-straight orientation with "well, you never know, you might change" isn't a practical or useful response; it suggests the responding person is processing asexuality as if it must be a passing phase. Sexual orientations are nothing but descriptions of patterns that have, so far in a person's life, been predictable. **Sexuality can be fluid, but**

there's no reason to point this out as a way to suggest someone can, will, or *should* change.

Heterosexual people don't have to add qualifiers to their orientation to be believed that they're heterosexual. Most people will not tell heterosexual people that they just need to meet the right gay person and their orientation will change. But LGBTQ folks and asexual folks do hear this—and, interestingly, sometimes asexual people hear this *from* LGBTQ folks as well as from heterosexual folks.

Orientation is a practical way to predict who one might be attracted to. It is based on past and present, and when the past and present have been consistent, there is no reason to believe that the future will be different—**nor is it practical to stake one's future relationships and lifestyles on that possibility**.

Asexual people aren't claiming they know, without a doubt, that they can't experience sexual attraction. But they're as qualified as anyone else to say they *don't*—that they haven't experienced it and aren't currently experienc-

> "I guess everyone's sexuality could change one day, but when people tell us 'maybe you haven't met the right person yet,' it seems painfully irrelevant—what about how we are right now? I'm A right now, and I always have been. (. . .) But even if I realize, in two days or two decades, that I'm secretly heterosexual, I will always support the A-Team."
>
> —ILY, *ASEXY BEAST*

ing it—and have every reason to believe they won't experience it in the future because of this. Most asexual people aren't interested in dedicating their lives to searching for a partner to change them. No one can assume asexual people are (or should be) hoping or trying to change themselves. **And they do not have an obligation to keep looking for a partner who can "wake up" their supposedly sleeping interest in sex.**

Sometimes the comments like "you haven't met the right person yet" sound like "Oh yeah? What about [insert hot celebrity]?"—as if the asexual person would have to admit that if it was Brad Pitt, they'd make an exception. [Author's note: For some reason, for my generation, it always seems to be Brad Pitt.] No, the asexual person doesn't find the movie star flavor of the month sexually attractive.

Sometimes people who say this believe asexual people aren't meeting enough sexy people in real life, but that a truly stunning specimen would flip even an asexual person's switch. Well, no. [Author's note: I've told multiple people that I'm not attracted to manliness at all, only to have them respond with "Yeah right,

> "I do not want anyone mistaking me for someone they can convert, coerce, or persuade. I don't want to be considered shy, inexperienced (and in need of a guiding hand), or sexually embryonic."
> —M. LeClerc, *Hypomnemata*

you would melt if [flavor of the month] walked in with his abs hanging out and demanded to ravish you." Why yes, I *can* say I wouldn't melt. I'd find that extremely creepy, actually, if a stranger walked into my house shirtless and expected me to respond positively. That may spoil the worldview of the hypothetical unbeliever, but I actually mean it when I say I'm not attracted to anyone. That includes Brad Pitt.]

Anyone hoping to understand an asexual friend or loved one should not go this route in encouraging asexual people to keep trying. Acknowledging one's asexuality doesn't constitute giving up on finding a partner or making a decision about one's future. It's just a description—a label the asexual person will wear until or unless it stops fitting, and there's a very good chance it will continue to fit. It shouldn't be understood or processed as a placeholder.

Is Asexuality a Religious Statement?

This question is caught up in how strongly virginity and abstinence are associated with purity and moral goodness. The easy answer is no—asexuality has nothing to do with religion. And considering that avoiding sex and supposedly triumphing over earthly desire implies that a person possesses the desire for sex in the first place, it wouldn't make any sense for a non-sex-desiring asexual person to claim abstention as a show of religious sacrifice.

In fact, some asexual people who *have* been raised in a religious or socially conservative atmosphere feel confused and alienated by the emphasis on "resisting" and "temptation." They may or may not feel lucky to have no trouble abstaining from sex, and they may or may not feel conflicted about why everyone presents avoiding sex as such a struggle. It's even happened that some religious authorities who praise chastity as a symbol of purity turn around and deny fellowship, turn down clergy status, or simply look down on a person who hasn't had to sacrifice to achieve it.

Also, since some of these circles stress waiting for marriage before having sex, some asexual people who desire marriage but not sex may fear what they'll be expected to do to satisfy the requirements of their religion. Even though sex before marriage is taught as a sin in some belief systems, refusing to have sex inside of a marriage can also be considered a failure to satisfy religious expectations. Asexual people from religious backgrounds may feel they have no option but to avoid all romantic relationships if they want to avoid being forced to submit to the marriage bed.

Some Christian scriptures mention lifelong celibacy being acceptable for those who do not desire sex,[13] while marriage is recommended for those who do desire sex.[14] With marriage being offered as the solution to the (supposed) problem of lust, those who may want to be chaste in a marriage may not be accepted. In Islam, though marriage is emphasized as expected, there is still room for celibacy, but similarly, it's recommended only for those who don't marry.[15] In traditional Judaism, propagation of the people is of primary importance;[16] some doctrines even say celibacy breaks religious law, since it constitutes failure to fulfill the divine command to have children.[17]

In philosophies that emphasize erasure of desire as a route to purity, such as Buddhism, innate lack of sexual "distraction" may be mistaken for a sign of enlightenment—or, conversely, may be regarded as *cheating* or *too easy*. And in Pagan philosophies that celebrate nature—especially those with fertility rites that symbolically and literally unite the masculine and the feminine—sex may be glorified and asexual people who refuse sex or don't feel comfortable with expressing themselves through sexual symbolism could be regarded as unable to fully participate. Even in mainstream, conservative, or strict religions, depending on the leader or the denomination of the belief system, sex is sometimes glorified (provided it's between married people) as being a gift from their deity and a holy expression.

It's commonly believed that conservative religious organizations would applaud abstinence (at least for unmarried folks), but some mainstream views about sex can be destructive to asexual people who receive them in a religious context. For instance, the same folks who call homosexuality unnatural because of religious beliefs also have a tendency to automatically frame heterosexuality as

---

13 "Now to the unmarried and the widows I say: It is good for them to stay unmarried, as I do. But if they cannot control themselves, they should marry, for it is better to marry than to burn with passion." (NIV: 1 Corinthians 7:8-9).

14 On why Paul, who remained celibate, recommends marriage for those who desire sex: "I say this as a concession, not as a command. I wish that all of you were as I am. But each of you has your own gift from God; one has this gift, another has that." (NIV: 1 Corinthians 7:6-7).

15 "[I]f one's healthful condition, integrity of heart, and peace of soul reside in celibacy then that is better for him, since these are things that are desired of marriage. If one can reach these without marriage then celibacy causes no harm." (*The Sustenance of the Hearts (Qut al-qulub)* —Abu Talib al-Makki)

16 "Be fruitful and multiply and fill the earth." (Bereshit 1:28)

17 "Every man is obligated to marry a woman in order to reproduce. Anyone who is not having children is as if they were killers." (*Shulhan Arukh*, Even Ha'Ezer 1:1)

natural—as the only natural sexuality. Living a life without heterosexual attraction may be regarded as unnatural from a religious point of view, and some religious leaders may even offend or alienate asexual believers by saying their orientation constitutes denial of a gift from their deity. They may pressure or shame asexual people for perceived or actual unwillingness to subscribe to traditional family arrangements because of their orientation; asexuality is certainly not the widely celebrated or preferred orientation that many outside these belief systems think it is.

There are, however, some belief systems and denominations of religions that are supportive of asexuality without misunderstanding it as a show of spiritual strength. Asexual people who want to practice their religion without receiving damaging messages about their orientation might consider looking at organizations that support tolerance, diversity, and individual choice in these matters. A congregation, religious leader, or denomination that vocally supports LGBTQ issues or emphasizes the importance of modern scientific or open-minded world views might be safe and healthy for a religious asexual person. There are interpretations of most faiths that will not condemn the orientation.

Unfortunately, some people have an immediate negative reaction to hearing about asexuality because they imagine asexual people believe themselves superior—that they must see themselves as having risen above supposedly animalistic urges for sex. So some may get defensive if they believe asexual people are making religious or moral statements by declaring their orientation. But most asexual people do not perceive sexual activity as an experience that sullies a person's goodness, and the orientation is not about abstaining so they can claim they are better than anyone else.

> "If asexuals are chaste, it's not usually because they hold it up as a virtue. It's because they would rather be chaste, regardless of whether or not they happen to think it is a virtue. I certainly do not regard chastity as a virtue; furthermore, like many other asexuals, I am not chaste. I find it really offensive to stuff these 'values' into my mouth and pretend that's what I asked for."
> —Tristan Miller, *Skeptic's Play*

Even outside of a religious context, saving oneself for marriage is a common show of devotion and honor—an abstention that garners respect from some people. Virginity is more commonly respected for women (until they get "too old," at which point they're pitied and mocked for not having sex), but people of all genders do sometimes hear "I admire that you're saving yourself!" from well-meaning folks. Asexuality isn't a means of saving oneself. Yet many will immediately assume that anyone who's not having sex has to be saving it for a particular type of relationship. Some asexual people may do this, just like some people of any orientation do this, but it is not "part of being asexual" as a rule.

Asexuality is not a behavior—it's a perspective on or experience of other people's attractiveness—so a person who comes out as asexual shouldn't be interpreted as though they are announcing a chastity vow.

Are Asexual People Going Through a Phase or Seeking Attention by Being Different?

"It's just a stage you're going through."

No one likes being dismissed as "following a fad" when they're expressing how they feel. It's true that sometimes people take a while to figure themselves out, of course. Some people do go through phases, and it shouldn't reflect poorly on anyone's opinion of asexuality if they've heard of or met a person who was initially mistaken in choosing that label (or discovered their orientation was fluid later in life).

The trouble with asexuality is that no one can prove a negative, so if it turns out a person is a late-blooming non-asexual person, that may externally look like asexuality before the blooming starts. That's not asexuality's fault, and it's also very frustrating (especially for young asexual people) if their friends and family react to their coming out by dismissing their feelings as nothing but a phase. Asexual teens also usually take longer than other people their age to identify their sexual orientation because they're encouraged to consider themselves late bloomers.

Asexual people shouldn't be told they'll "grow out of it." The prevailing asexual community narratives encourage people of all ages to stay very in touch with themselves while understanding their sexuality and to not deliberately squash or avoid sexual feelings if they do become part of their experiences later on. For the most part, continued identity exploration is respected, though here and there elitists will suggest that the questioning members of asexual communities might make asexuality look bad. Teens shouldn't be automatically subjected to doubt because of their age, especially since *if they really are asexual*, they're figuring that out about the same time other people are figuring out that they find others sexually attractive, and they're probably wondering what's wrong with them.

There is nothing to be gained from dismissing a young asexual person as necessarily facing a future "maturation" into a more common sexual orientation. There's no purpose in telling a young person who feels they are asexual that they will grow out of it, nor is it helpful to "reassure" them that they will find a partner and stop being asexual. It's important for them to know that asexuality is a valid conclusion—that they don't have to grow up thinking something is wrong with them because they aren't interested in what their friends are interested in. Those who would like to avoid making asexual young people feel inferior should not say any of these things.

Occasional critics say they used to be asexual but outgrew it or that they knew someone who used to be asexual but stopped being asexual. This isn't relevant, because one person's experience doesn't invalidate another's. Some perspectives from people who thought they were asexual and realized it wasn't true are interesting, though—for instance, sometimes transgender people who identified as asexual before transition find sexual attraction developing in their post-transition lives. And sometimes people explore their attraction experiences and intimacy preferences only to find they no longer fit under the asexual umbrella.

Other critics sometimes say asexual people need to try sex before they can determine whether they like it. This is levied at younger asexual people more often because it's commonly assumed they have not had sex and couldn't have the perspective to understand whether they'd like it. Society's norms more or less expect everyone to have had sex by a certain age, and asexual teens are often spoken to as if their eventual sexual experiences are inevitable. Asexual people shouldn't be told they'll grow up, have sex, and change their minds, no matter what age they are.

"You're not asexual; you're just socially awkward."

It's true that most people go through an "awkward" stage sometime in their lives, and that for most people, that awkward stage comes somewhere during puberty. But for most teens, their first sexual attractions are compelling enough to inspire them to pursue partners anyway—especially since many young people are all socially awkward at the same time and can find comfort in bumbling through it together in their first experiences.

And yes, while being socially awkward can inhibit someone's chances to socialize (including with potential partners), it's unlikely someone would use asexuality as an excuse to avoid these relationships. There are plenty of reasons teens might not be ready to pursue partners, but responding to their identity with "no, it's not that you don't *want* anyone; it's that you *can't get* anyone" certainly isn't going to help their awkwardness. Confidence in one's approach does have something to do with successful relationships and making connections, but asexuality is a description of how someone feels, not what they do.

"But seriously. Stop trying to seem special!"

Asexual people are often accused of identifying as asexual for attention. However, the kind of attention they get for it is often negative, so those who are only looking to have their specialness praised are unlikely to use the label for long. For most asexual people, "you just want to be special" is a particularly disappointing reaction. Most of them aren't yearning for any kind of special status; they just want to be listened to, judged to be reasonable, and allowed to go on with their lives without facing pity or harassment. Sharing something personal about themselves only to be labeled an attention-seeking faker may lead them to avoid sharing personal information in the future.

Some people do have inauthentic reasons for identifying as asexual, and it's always possible someone might be using a sexual orientation (any sexual orientation) to get attention or run with a cause. But it isn't helpful at all to suggest that this is the case for any particular person. Those who claim an asexual-identified person is only looking for attention will be likely to lose the asexual person's trust.

Sometimes asexuality awareness efforts are criticized due to fear of "recruiting." Some people—particularly abusive authority figures, sex therapists who have not done proper research, and people who lack empathy—believe awareness about asexuality is *dangerous*. Some have said they oppose awareness because it might catch on like a fad and encourage people to ignore their sexual feelings or embrace abstinence rather than work through kinks or non-heteronormative sexual issues that might be disturbing them.[18]

These folks believe that if we pass on knowledge about this orientation existing, some people might label themselves prematurely and stop looking for their "real" sexuality. They seem to ignore that asexual people can be (and usually are) damaged by lack of awareness about their orientation. When these people advocate silencing this dialogue on behalf of people who might otherwise mislabel themselves and experience pain and confusion, it's clear they only care about this kind of pain if non-asexual people are being hurt. No sympathy comes for asexual people who are forced through lack of language and knowledge to choose some other ill-fitting label and miserably attempt to embody it.

People don't decide they're asexual on a whim once they hear it's an option. They usually find a word for what they feel and something clicks for them, resulting in profound gratefulness and relief. **People who are asexual typically**

---

18 "It looks like such a dodge from outside. I know from experience, and I know from giving people advice about their sex lives for thirteen years, a lot of people are deeply conflicted about their desires, and a lot of people are really conflicted about their sexual orientations, and for a lot of these people it'd be easier just to not have a sexual orientation. It'd be a great escape to say 'oh, I'm not gay, I'm not a lesbian, I'm not bi, or my heterosexuality's so disturbing to me because my kinks are this and this and this, that I'm just asexual, I'm NOTHING.'" —Dan Savage, as quoted in the documentary *(A)sexual*. (Tucker, 2011)

struggle for years trying to find some indication of what's wrong with them or whether anyone else feels the way they do. And if they enter an asexual community and begin having nuanced discourse about intimacy and connection, they aren't encouraged to put a lid on further self-growth. They're encouraged to explore and explain their identity for better personal and interpersonal understanding.

> "I have definitely thought about my own sexuality (or lack thereof, depending on your perspective) since getting involved in the ace community more than I did in the preceding two decades of my life combined."
> —QUEENIE, THE ASEXUAL AGENDA

These communities discuss romance, sex, relationships, and different forms of attraction in such detail that it certainly wouldn't be practical to run falsely to asexuality in the hopes that it would make one's life simpler. When asexual-identified people are dismissed with phrases like "I bet you got this idea from the Internet" or "so is this what the cool kids are doing now?" it's even more isolating and harmful. Especially once they've found a community on the Internet and finally figured out they weren't alone. To finally have this kind of revelation only to be invalidated is hurtful and disappointing.

Most asexual people were struggling for understanding before finding a community, and their rarity makes finding each other offline very unlikely. The Internet is the only option for many if they want to connect with others like themselves. But that doesn't mean they got the idea from the Internet; this would be like asking if people got the idea to try sex from watching porn online.

Asexual people feel asexual regardless of whether they have a word for it, and though increased awareness about asexuality might lead to some incorrect or premature labeling, awareness efforts are still very important. [Author's note: As a young asexual person, I wrote essays about being "nonsexual" and posted them online long before the main asexual network based around *AVEN* was created, and many other asexual people were independently inventing words to describe themselves before they found others.]

There's also the reversal of this: people think asexual people have suddenly become gung-ho about wanting everyone to know about their asexuality, while they think it really doesn't need awareness efforts. A common reaction sounds like "Well what's the point? It's not like people are getting asexual-bashed." And beyond some cases of "corrective" rape, overall no, asexual people usually aren't attacked physically over their orientation. (And they're grateful for that.) But anyone who thinks the only reason to raise awareness is to prevent physical violence is wrong.

Mostly, asexual people would like to foster an experience of coming out that doesn't require a subsequent thirty- to forty-minute education

> "Even if we feel positive about our asexuality, the onus is always on the asexual to prove ourselves. (. . .) People tell us our orientation is too confusing or unusual to bother with understanding. It's not hard to start believing that they may be right, and that there is some inherent problem with the 'difficulty' of asexuality and, therefore, with us."
>
> —ILY, *ASEXY BEAST*

session during which they must defend and explain the existence of their orientation. Asexual people would like to stop hearing that people like them need to be "fixed." **Awareness is needed for many reasons, and a non-asexual person viewing the issue as unimportant and personally irrelevant does not invalidate asexual people's need to educate on the subject.**

Wouldn't Asexual People Be Lonely All the Time?

This is another example of projection. "If I'm lonely without a partner, everyone else without a partner must be lonely too! Even if they say otherwise!"

Very few people believe the only meaningful relationships have to be sexual. It's true that the institution of the couple is upheld nearly everywhere as a building block of family and society. And it's true that most people consider their significant others to be the most important people in their lives or their best friends. There's nothing wrong with that. But it makes no sense to say asexual people—even those who don't date—must therefore have no one important, no one significant, no best friend in their lives.

Most people want to connect with others in some way, but everyone has different ways of doing so. Some people believe those who reach out in different ways, with different effects, must be hollow inside, missing something essential in life, secretly wishing for this connection that they supposedly lack. "They

> "I'm not great at the whole dating thing, but I'm still a human being and I crave emotional intimacy. If I don't date, I have to figure out how to get those connections through an alternate way, and if I do date, I have to figure out how to either connect to other asexual people (difficult) or negotiate expectations that romantic relationships be sexual relationships, too."
>
> —SCIATRIX, *THE ASEXUAL AGENDA*

don't have sex! How depressing is that? They must have terrible, empty lives." Happily, that perception of how asexual people feel is a myth.

Most asexual people have no particular problems forging and holding onto the relationships that matter most to them. Most of their partnered relationships work a little differently, and those who don't form partnered relationships value different interaction experiences with their peers. Most people feel lonely sometimes, but asexual people don't automatically carry around a pit that can never be filled. Many have active social lives and can forge satisfying, intimate relationships of all types.

Some, especially those who are introverts, may seem "lonely" if they spend most of their time alone, but preferring solitude isn't the same as being lonely. Some have different emotional needs and really don't crave intimate or particularly emotional connection with others as much as they're expected to. Being aromantic, asexual, and alone most of the time is not a sign of pathology; plenty of well-adjusted people are most satisfied with their own company and may not crave social attention or go out of their way to spend time with others. It's just one more perfectly valid way to be.

"So you're just going to be a cat lady, I get it."

No, you don't.

The "cat lady" comment is often dropped on people (mostly women) who don't want partners. Putting aside the fact that many asexual people do want partners—even if some don't want sex with said partners—calling people who want to remain single "cat ladies" is usually intended to pigeonhole them as pathetic singletons who hoard cats to assuage their loneliness. (Though there's nothing wrong with loving your cats!) No one likes when others assume they're going to spend their lives mourning their horrible, lonely fate—not to mention that if a person *was* lonely, that loneliness would be nothing to mock.

However, no one should suggest someone's choices based on orientation are going to lead to an unenviable, desperate life. Asexual people will often react to these assumptions by mistrusting and withdrawing from the people who voice them, and it's possible that repeatedly subjecting them to comments about their supposedly terrible lives will push them toward becoming despondent and self-conscious.

Similarly, sometimes asexual people are assumed to be depressed if they don't make sexual and/or romantic connections. Depression, or medication associated with treatment, does sometimes decrease sexual interest and sexual arousal ability.[19] That doesn't mean it's the other way around. People don't automatically

---

19 "Studies have demonstrated an association between depression and diminished libido in addition to sexual dysfunction that can occur as a side effect of many antidepressants." (Miller & Hunt, 2003)

have a mood disorder if they don't pursue or enjoy sex. **People who are both asexual and depressed do exist, but treating the depression doesn't make them attracted to people if they are asexual.**

Are Asexual People Repressed, Boring, or Dispassionate?

"But . . . then what do you *do* all day?"

Folks who say this clearly consider sexual attraction—and the relationships that often grow out of it—to be central to their lives and allow these relationships to take up a great deal of their time and attention. Without this focus, many people can't imagine what their lives would be like and imagine asexual people to simply have a void there. The truth is that most people have passions . . . which they pursue, well, passionately. If a person is interested in sex and sexual relationships, they pursue them and give them a lot of attention. Asking what an asexual person could be *doing* all day is condescending and misleading.

Chasing or enjoying sexual passion is not the only way to express a lust for life. Some think asexual people are deliberately sacrificing or avoiding "the good things in life," or must be hiding the desire for these activities deep inside, where even they might not acknowledge them. Those who misunderstand asexuality as abstention for the purpose of self-denial (possibly for some higher purpose) often believe asexual people just don't know how to have fun. For people who—again—cannot empathize or refuse to, it's impossible to imagine sex as unappealing. **Sex is appealing to *them*; therefore, they insist sex is objectively appealing, and those who are not chasing it must feel unsatisfied.** If they were asked to give up sex—or any other passion—they'd definitely feel like it was a sacrifice and feel a loss in their lives. It's much easier for them to label an asexual person a boring straight-edger or a repressed killjoy than it is to imagine that not having sex is one natural lifestyle for a person who isn't attracted to other people that way.

> "(W)hen we asexuals are expressing this lack of contentment, it's not actually because we wish we were sexual people who could have a sexual relationship. We simply want a relationship where we are loved and respected for who we are, and that is sadly difficult to find. One is a discontent with identity; the other is a discontent with the practical negotiation of that identity in the world."
>
> —M. LeClerc, *Hypomnemata*

And then some people believe that without sexual interest, a person would just be lifeless. They compare lack of interest in sex to a lack of interest in eating or breathing. Asked to imagine or comprehend asexual people, their response is to call up a zombie being with no juice, and the idea is horrifying and alienating to them. **It's hard for them to relate to asexual people if they believe sexual attraction is a driving, central, essential force in a person's life and asexual people have none.**

But it isn't as if lack of sexual desire or sexual attraction is the same as lack of desires of any kind. Asexual people don't automatically lack motivation and energy or any vital "juice." People who look at asexual people as though they must be zombies or robots are probably looking at them as a concept rather than as people.

An interesting reversal of this question comes when some suggest asexual people must get so much done in their lives only because they "have so much time on their hands." As discussed earlier, people tend to spend their time pursuing what they love, and asexual people aren't different in that respect. It isn't as though everyone in the world is assigned a time-management pie chart with a wedge meant to be dedicated to "relationships and sex" and therefore asexual and/or aromantic people get an advantage in all the other categories. They don't have a blank space they have to try desperately to fill with activities. They don't lack a necessary motivating factor in personal passion. And they don't, as a group, have less lust for life than anyone else.

Aren't Asexual People Being Awfully Selfish? Isn't an Asexual Person a Tease?

"What a waste."

Yes, asexual people hear this if they're not open to sexual relationships. Some will state an asexual person is "a waste" if a potential sexual partner doesn't get to experience them in the bedroom. They're an attractive body with the potential for lovemaking and they're just *wasting* it. How bothersome it is that their personal inclinations and desires get in the way of their bodies being enjoyed by someone who wants them!

The phrasing of the sentiments above are absurd exaggerations, but their essence is frequently communicated to asexual people. It may sound ridiculous—because it is—but it is nevertheless a common reaction, usually unthinkingly blurted without regard for how dehumanizing statements like these are. A person who abstains from sex isn't "a waste" just because sex is possible but avoided.

Many people's bodies also have the capacity to become Olympic gymnasts with lots of hard work and practice. Are people who don't pursue the Olympics a waste? Plenty of attractive people aren't models. Is that a waste?

It's not selfish whatsoever for asexual people to live lifestyles that correspond to their wishes. **Calling an asexual person *selfish* for not engaging in sex suggests they are denying other people something they deserve.** It's saying asexual people owe other people sex just by virtue of having a body that could execute it. It's much more "selfish" to claim asexual people are obligated to offer sex *against their own wishes*.

When someone is attracted to an asexual person and the asexual person cannot or does not reciprocate the interest, the asexual person sometimes gets called "a tease" or gets accused of "leading people on." This, of course, is not unique to asexual people; many

> "Asexuality is a free pass out of exactly zero of the thousands of ways the patriarchy polices female sexuality. (. . .) That I enjoy being attractive, without wanting to attract anyone and without being attracted to anyone, puts me squarely in that illogical category known as 'being a tease,' just like millions of other women who dare to do something for themselves rather than for a male audience."
> —AYDAN SELBY, *THE ASEXUAL AGENDA*

people have this experience of being on the receiving end of unwanted romantic or sexual attention, and they may respond to it by declaring disinterest. This rejection is often met with a suggestion that the recipient did something wrong by not reciprocating the interest. This accusation suggests asexual people's sexual orientation is about others, and it's not.

"Well that's awfully frigid of you."

This statement and others like it are often thrown at people—usually women—if they dare to make themselves sexually unavailable for any reason, so asexual people hear it pretty often. Asexual people are not frigid, cold, unfeeling, or (again) failing to deliver something they owe someone. It's invoked especially often to shame people in relationships who do not want to engage in sex or do not want to engage in sex often enough to please their partner(s).

"I bet you just get off on playing hard-to-get."

It's inevitable that some people will interpret "I'm asexual" as a game. Equating asexual people's lack of sexual attraction to others with "playing" (expecting the end result to involve being "gotten") strongly suggests that *yes* means "yes" and *no* means "keep trying." *No* should be taken seriously and respected.

And, of course, romantic asexual people especially get to hear "you're so selfish!" because if they happen to be in a sexless relationship, they're perceived as cruelly withholding sex from a partner who deserves it. "Don't you think you should let them get a *real* partner?" is a common statement thrown at romantic asexual people by those who think sex is part of any meaningful romantic partnership, usually coming from people who misunderstand a sexless romance as indistinguishable from a friendship.

Ultimately, everyone who wants a relationship has dealbreakers. Some would say it's a dealbreaker if a partner expects them to have sex. Some would say it's a dealbreaker if a partner won't have sex (or won't have a minimum amount of sex). **Lack of sex is *not*, however, a dealbreaker for *all* people who experience sexual attraction, especially since there are ways to have a satisfactory sex life without the asexual partner(s) participating in sex.** Implying that the asexual person is cruel for withholding sex makes no more sense than referring to the asexual person's partner(s) as cruel for wanting sex. If either situation truly is a dealbreaker, the partners will just have to break the deal. Otherwise, they should be trusted to negotiate their own relationship without anyone accusing the asexual partner(s) of spoiling it.

What about asexual people who are very sexually appealing but unavailable? Are they really "teases"? Say, if they don't want sex, why the false advertising? Why try to look attractive? Why wear nice clothes or care about aesthetic standards if anyone who propositions them is going to get shut down? What a cruel thing to do!

First off, people who are married or in serious relationships and are monogamous—in other words, off the market—aren't obligated to immediately do everything in their power to look disgusting. There is *so* much more that goes into looking aesthetically pleasing in our society besides that which has to do with sex. Many people feel more confident when they feel they look good, and even those who are not particularly interested in physical appearance will still usually care about hygiene. It's inaccurate to claim that looking good only functions to attract mates or that those who don't want mates are sending out misleading signals.

People do not present themselves according to socially acceptable aesthetic guidelines solely to attract mates or keep existing mates happy. Most people do not make a conscious decision to avoid hygiene or flattering clothes based on a belief that they will not see potential mates or existing mates that day. Appearance is used to judge people for many other reasons besides sexual interest.

This also is aimed at women and those perceived as women much more often than any other gender and is sometimes framed in a way that sounds like shaming: namely, if a woman doesn't go out of her way to avoid someone being attracted to her (*or* she does wear flattering clothes or makeup), she owes people who are attracted to her some kind of follow-through. If she replies that she's not interested, she is perceived as reneging on an understood contract. No one should tell anyone that they're doing something unfair or inconsistent if they look nice but they refuse to consent to sex.

Don't Asexual People Need to Procreate?

"Then what's your purpose in life?"

Some people have a hard time imagining how a person could want anything out of life or have any passion for anything if they aren't interested in getting a partner, enjoying a partnered life, or having children. Suggesting a person has no purpose if they aren't interested in procreation is very dismissive and offensive.

"But if everyone was like you, you know there'd be no more babies, right?"

Reproduction is completely irrelevant to a conversation about asexuality. Some asexual people still want to reproduce (and can do so), but beyond that, *asexual people are not advocating "conversion" to asexuality for everyone else.* Clearly procreative sex is the most popular way children are brought into the world. It does not mean that every single person on the planet must have children.

Many societies generally accept birth control usage without attacking users as unnatural. People beyond the reproductive age who want to have sex aren't unnatural. People who are congenitally infertile or became so through surgery aren't unnatural for continuing to have sex, though some might treat them as if they have a debilitating condition or may disapprove of those who choose sterilization without having children first. But asexual people hear "that's unnatural!" constantly. And even though babies clearly aren't at the root of this accusation, "But what about the babies?!" has become a rallying cry for those who want to tell asexual people there's something intrinsically wrong with them. Even if we intellectually decided not to have kids, our bodies should still want to, right? Why, it's part of being alive!

The species isn't about to die out due to low birth rate. There is no reason to harass asexual people if they fail to reproduce just because reproduction is important to the continuation of the species. Variants have always existed in every species, and if they do not contribute to the destruction of the population, the variants keep popping up. From an extremely narrow biological perspective, an individual organism is not successful if it cannot grow to adulthood and reproduce. But since the species does not define its overall "success" simply through reproduction—and since nurturing and protecting other members of the species is also necessary for the species' survival regardless of whether an individual reproduces—there is no need to chastise asexual people for failure to reproduce as though they are traitors to the species.

Many asexual people still want children. Many opt for the same types of procedures that are available to partners who can't procreate with each other and people who can't or don't want to create or carry children. And some asexual people are willing to have sex for procreative purposes, just like one doesn't have to enjoy the process of IVF implantation to be willing to undergo it for purposes of getting a child. Sexual attraction isn't necessary to go through with sex. Sometimes the desire for a child is stronger than the disinterest or possible revulsion that some asexual people feel toward sex.

> "Motherhood isn't natural, 'amazing,' or inevitable for all women. It's viable for men to have other outlets of creation—novels, music, scientific discoveries, and it shouldn't be any different for women. I don't think having biological kids is out of the question for me—maybe a physical struggle will be preferable to a bureaucratic struggle if and when I do decide I want kids. I can guess why 'your own kids' are so important to people . . . sort of . . . but I don't feel it viscerally. Maybe I never will, and that's just fine."
>
> —Ily, *Asexy Beast*

To sum up, a) "but sex makes babies!" is neither a compelling reason to have sex nor a revelation for asexual people; b) asexual people aren't a threat to others' sex or baby-making; c) the world population does not need a boost; and d) asexual people can have babies if they decide they want them.

Do Asexual People Hate Sex or People Who Have Sex?

Asexual people don't automatically think everyone else is an animalistic lower life-form. Asexual people don't all think non-asexual people or their activities are disgusting. Identifying as asexual doesn't include a moral judgment against sexual activities. Asexual people aren't identifying as asexual as a way of saying they're better than others.

Most asexual people support everyone's freedom to pursue sex responsibly however they like—as long as *not* pursuing sex is also considered acceptable. Normally their only negative feelings on the subject are directed toward those who won't stop harassing them to pursue and value sex the same as most of the rest of the world. Some asexual people might recognize that critics think they're helping, but sometimes asexual people's annoyance toward or criticism of people who try to "help" them this way can be misinterpreted as disgust for or hate toward people who experience sexual attraction or sex itself. That's not the case.

The asexual population does contain occasional elitists who will look down on others for what they believe and practice about sex, but that is just as likely to come from people who do experience sexual attraction or do have sex but make different choices about it than whoever they're judging. It's not inherent to the asexual "lifestyle" that they want to shame people for having sex, or for liking it, or for being sexually attracted to others. **And while many asexual people can't understand that drive everyone else talks about, it doesn't mean they're judging everyone else negatively for it.**

Actually, some asexual people celebrate sex—up to and including engaging in it themselves despite lack of sexual attraction. Some asexual people write stories or produce art depicting sexual situations and/or nudity. Some asexual people have no problem with consuming media that contains sexual content. They do not have to be attracted to other people to appreciate or create positive portrayals of these relationships.

This can be especially difficult to explain if an asexual artist does create sexually explicit material, because people want to know whether they're creating this because they secretly desire it. Or they might reverse the issue and suggest asexual people have no business creating this media—or that they can't be good at it—if they don't have personal experience. **What artists choose to make art about has absolutely no bearing on what they're attracted to or what they might want to experience themselves.** Art *can* be used to express personal desires, but no one should assume someone *must* be doing so if that person depicts experiences or images contrary to personally expressed desires, and no one should use a person's artwork or subject matter to invalidate claims.

Asexual artists cannot be restricted to creating media that is devoid of sex. Asexual artists know and accept that most people are attracted sexually to others, so if they want to write realistic books or movies, they generally have to create at least some of their subjects with that dimension attached to them.

Some asexual people make sexually explicit statements, have "dirty" minds, or laugh at sexual humor. This can cause some bewildered observers to protest, "Wait, I thought you were *asexual*. You're supposed to think sex is gross or dirty. If you're laughing at that joke or want to see that movie, how can you be asexual?" Appreciation of jokes, language, and sexual content does not indicate a brain primed for sexual attraction. Asexual people are just as varied on this point as the general population; some appreciate sexual humor or make sex jokes or can pick up on sexual undertones, and doing so does not undermine their claim to being asexual.

Similarly, no one should assume it's necessary to censor themselves in front of asexual people. If anyone—asexual or not—asks to avoid certain topics, it's best to respect them. But it's unlikely that casual mentions of sex will disgust someone's asexual friends and family, and *explicit* discussions of sex are probably something most people should get the okay for when having them with anyone. Asexual people are not disgusted by the fact that others have sex (at least, not as a rule), and they don't need language filters to protect their supposedly virgin ears. If a person wants to know how a particular asexual person feels about this subject, they should ask instead of assume. Taking it for granted that asexual people would be horrified has a "let's not talk about this in front of the children" feeling and may seem condescending to asexual people.

Please note that while some asexual people proudly associate with the sex-positive movement, there are also plenty of asexual people who may not hate sex, but do not identify as sex positive. Some feel that sex is something they just don't want to be involved in or be exposed to, and quite a lot of people—including people who aren't asexual—have plenty to say that's critical of sexualized culture. These perspectives are also valued, and it's not elitist or shaming to suggest taking a good look at the damaging messages frequently hammered home by pervasive and compulsory sexuality in society. Some folks just want nothing to do with it, and some others would resent being told that sex positivity is required.

There are sex-neutral, sex-nonjudgmental, and sex-averse people in the world who are alienated by (or at least not automatically supportive of) the overtly sexual nature of some sex-positive rhetoric and outreach, and this attitude does not make them anti-sexual or elitist. It just means they don't personally relate and don't want to be forced into celebrations of sex as if to prove they're not against it either.

Occasionally, asexual people (especially those just coming to terms with their identity) celebrate their asexuality in misguided ways, and so unfortunately there is sex shaming, sexuality shaming, sex drive shaming, promiscuity shaming, and sex-worker shaming in the community sometimes. Some asexual people engage in this behavior as a way of striking back at a culture they feel has hurt them, rejecting the shame they've been subjected to for failing to conform to compulsory sexuality and "reclaiming" their pride through moralistic claims. Most asexual people who go through this phase eventually realize they don't have to attack sex for their own asexuality to be acceptable.

However, sometimes this anger and elitism is interpreted as the reason behind their asexuality. They're just angry at sex, some say, or angry at being left out. The asexuality itself is interpreted as a pretense to cover an asexual person's frustration or hatred, and it's assumed that they'd start feeling sexual attraction in a more normative fashion if they'd just stop being so angry. This is yet another way asexuality can be invalidated: if it can be recategorized as a lack of interest that grows out of a maladaptive attitude toward sex, asexuality doesn't have to be considered as an orientation.

Angry, elitist, and sex-shaming asexual people do exist, but their attitudes are not representative of the community, nor are these attitudes part of what defines them as asexual. Asexual communities often challenge their members' expressions of elitism and shaming toward non-asexual people where they occur.

Should Asexual People Get Therapy to Be Fixed?

"But orgasms are wonderful!" "But I have such a connection with my wife when we make love!" "But you're missing out on so much!" "How could you not be curious about this and want it for yourself?" "If you have no interest in the best thing in the world, you should really get help. . . ."

Some asexual people like orgasms and pursue them in various ways available to them, and they still identify as asexual because arousal and satisfaction are not sexual attraction. Also, asexual people tend to hear a lot of "I'm sorry I'm having so much trouble with this, but you see, it's just that I'm a *very sexual person!*" Followed by stories about how satisfying sex is. **The problem is that telling asexual people how great sex is smacks of talking down to them—like they are missing something vital and are deserving of pity.**

Most asexual people don't react to others talking about sex with stories about how great asexuality is. Abstinent asexual people could theoretically go on for hours about how great their lives are without having to worry about sexual escapades, and non-partner-desiring asexual people can brag all day about how they don't have to worry about all the ins and outs of the dating game. It still wouldn't be right for them to say "Shouldn't you get therapy to help you see how blissful this existence is?"

"But I just want you to be happy."

Most people understand that imposing their own desires on other people against those people's will is not about making *those* people happy. People who say this, or do this, are communicating that asexual people don't understand happiness and can't actually be content. Everyone should trust them to describe their own feelings, not attempt to impose their own. One thing that tends to make asexual people *un*happy is that other people feel the need to try to fix them, and it does cause stress.

If someone has trouble understanding how it could be wrong to encourage an abstinent asexual person to "open" to sexual experiences, that person should think about how they feel when they're offered unsolicited advice to an end they aren't interested in. Like if the waiter doesn't believe someone will like the meal they ordered and repeatedly insists that they should try *his* favorite dish (ultimately bringing it and charging them for it). **No one should badger an asexual person to change and say it's for the sake of *their* happiness. Those who won't stop trying to change content asexual people are usually much more upset about the situation than the asexual people are.**

As for whether asexual people need a counselor for anything sex-related that should be "fixed" . . . first off, strangers and acquaintances shouldn't bring up another person's mental health in a casual conversation. Secondly, this suggests asexual people should be trying to figure out what's "wrong" with them and working through trying to "fix" themselves so that they will either want sex or tolerate it. So they can be "normal." People who aren't straight have sometimes had to deal with this as well, though nowadays it's less likely that a gay, bisexual, polysexual, or pansexual person's decision to go to a mental health professional will lead immediately to "let's figure out what stopped you from being straight and try to reverse it."

Unfortunately, the outward "symptoms" of asexuality could still be considered a mental disorder in the *Diagnostic and Statistical Manual of Mental Disorders,*[20] and sometimes mental health professionals *do* believe the asexuality is a symptom even if the asexual person in question is getting help for something unrelated to that. **If a physical or mental health practitioner is not informed about asexuality, they could easily misdiagnose an asexual patient and fail to help at best or actively damage the person at worst** (all at the expense of the asexual person's time, money, and well-being).

"But I'm just trying to help you."

It doesn't feel like "help" if someone is pushing their own philosophy on someone else. Chances are, if someone has declared that they're asexual, they like themselves that way and they aren't going to be enticed to "change" because someone keeps expressing how concerned they are. This is especially suspicious for those who are not particularly nosy about any other aspect of the asexual person's health. If someone develops a fixation with whether an asexual person's

---

20 Hypoactive Sexual Desire Disorder: "Persistently or recurrently deficient (or absent) sexual/erotic thoughts or fantasies and desire for sexual activity." (American Psychiatric Association, 2013)

sex life looks enough like their own out of pure *concern* for their *health and happiness*, it seems odd they're not concerned with other aspects of the person's health. Perhaps if someone's really concerned about health, they should also be asking for updates on their bowel movements or monitoring their water intake. (Anybody who's asking these questions and is not a medical professional doing it in a medical context, please stop being creepy.)

"Well, are you sure you're actually asexual? Have you been diagnosed?"

Some people think asexual people can't actually be asexual unless a doctor has certified it. This is the only way some people can accept that something unusual is real, but doctors can't diagnose a sexual orientation. No one is diagnosed as straight by a doctor. It won't show up on a blood test or be confirmed by a brain scan. It is *supposed* to be subjective.

And on the subject of doctors, be advised that there isn't a pill to fix asexuality either. There is a pill for erectile dysfunction and/or medical interventions to result in increased libido, but as mentioned before, sex drive is not sexual attraction and nobody who's being supportive should suggest asexual people need to be medicated for asexuality.

The diagnosable disorder hypoactive sexual desire disorder sounds a little like asexuality on the outside; it's defined as "persistently or recurrently deficient (or absent) sexual/erotic thoughts or fantasies and desire for sexual activity."[21] For a diagnosis to be made, the current *Diagnostic and Statistical Manual of Mental Disorders* stipulates that the sufferer must be troubled by the symptoms. However, a previous version of the *DSM* allowed patients to be diagnosed with HSDD if it caused "interpersonal difficulty," and some have said if this causes friction between an asexual person and a partner, it also counts as "marked distress." Because of this (and a few other criticisms), this definition of HSDD has been criticized, and arguments were made in favor of recognizing asexuality as a sexual orientation in the fifth edition of the *Diagnostic and Statistical Manual of Mental Disorders*.[22] An exception for asexuality is now specifically mentioned, which should function as a heads-up for not only mental health professionals, but also for those who try to mimic them in "diagnosing" others.

Those who want to be supportive of asexual people should avoid telling them to look for a different way to approach their sexuality and their relationships. If someone is unhappy with themselves, it's their responsibility to change it, and unsolicited advice in this area is unwelcome.

---

21 Diagnostic Code 302.71. (American Psychiatric Association, 2013)
22 "Asexuality raises questions concerning the role of 'personal distress' in defining sexual desire problems." (Prause & Graham, 2007)

However, if they do want to pursue therapy or psychological counseling, asexual people can sometimes benefit. If an asexual person wants to see a counselor or mental health professional for a reason that might involve disclosing their sexual orientation, they should do some homework on their therapists and possibly come prepared to educate them. Sometimes professionals who have a background in LGBTQ and/or gender subjects can be more open to respecting asexual clients' orientation, but in this field, ignorance and invalidation are disturbingly common. If interviewing them first is possible, it is recommended.

An asexual person can be most comfortable in therapy if they know their sexual identity is accepted and will be fostered, not suspected as a symptom or treated as an illness to cure. Asexual people can ask their therapists to consult the current version of the *Diagnostic and Statistical Manual of Mental Disorders* (the *DSM-5*) and point out that asexuality is considered an exception to sexual arousal and desire disorders, and they may benefit from bringing in recent scientific research papers for their therapists to read. (Some research links are provided in Part Six of this book.) This helps signal that other medical professionals are taking asexuality seriously and they might want to do some independent research on the topic themselves if they want to be in the best position to treat an asexual client.

That said, pursuing therapy or counseling should be consensual; no one should pressure or make demands of an asexual person to go to a professional and "get fixed."

Aren't Asexual People So Lucky to Have Simple, Uncomplicated Lives Without Sex?

As is probably clear by now, asexual people's lives are far from uncomplicated. It's true that sexual relationships and partnered relationships add complications and stress to life, and sometimes when these stressors feel overwhelming, some might idealize those they perceive as free from these pressures. Mustn't their lives be so idyllic and carefree? They probably have as few problems as little children without the adult worries of sexual relationships and pressures hanging over their heads, right? Well, not exactly.

Asexual people who want partners have their own hoops to jump through, trying to negotiate atypical relationships that are anything but simple. They face the rarity of asexual partners versus the difficulty of compromising with non-asexual partners.

Non-partner-desiring asexual people, conversely, have to face a world that tells them their happiness as a singleton is erratic, unnatural, and alien, which often leads to those in their lives pressuring them (sometimes violently) to accept romantic and sexual attention. Aromantic and non-partner-desiring asexual people are often treated as though there's something deeply wrong with them, and people who present themselves as potential partners sometimes refuse to process these folks as unavailable since they're not "taken" or partnered. When their friendships are their most precious relationships, they are often dropped or demoted in importance if their partner-desiring friends get significant others, and they sometimes struggle with feeling like they can never be important enough to anyone.

Asexual people live in a world that defines the way they pursue intimacy as aberrant and often treats them poorly because of it. **Finessing relationships of any kind is difficult for those whose situation is considered inconceivable, worthy of interrogation, pathological, or in need of rehabilitation.**

Furthermore, asexual people's feelings are as nuanced and their lives as full as anyone else's. Romance, partnership, and sex are not the only adult experiences that make maturity a more complicated place than childhood. Still, some people feel that these definitive re-

> "For a long time I thought I was aromantic. I was looking at the translation of romance the world was showing me and I thought, 'I don't want that.' It took me a while to realize that just because I didn't want *that*—dinner dates and kissing in movie theaters—didn't mean I didn't want *something*. I had to reprogram myself, so to speak, and re-create what romance and relationships meant to me, not what they were supposed to mean."
>
> —AUDACIOUS ACE, *ASEXUALITY UNABASHED*

lationships require a huge amount of time and attention, and often the pursuit or the negotiation of relationships is so time-consuming, exhausting, and frustrating—sometimes with little payoff. Since some asexual people don't have to deal with it at all and many asexual people don't have to deal with it in the same way, the situation sometimes inspires people who have these problems to naively say, "I sure wish I was asexual. My life would be so much easier." Well, hypothetical person, you know not what you wish.

Many asexual people feel they are part of a misunderstood group. If someone says they wish they were asexual, they don't know what they're asking for, just like asexual people wouldn't know what they'd be asking for if they said they wished they could stop being asexual. An asexual person becoming sexually attracted to others would bring on many new problems, surely; the asexual person would be exposed to all sorts of unforeseen and difficult-to-process aspects of relationships. The reverse is also true.

Asexual people have to navigate relationships differently, and they have to interact with the world despite living inside a sex-focused culture they often can't relate to. It's condescending if a non-asexual person tells an asexual person that they wish they were asexual because one of their problems would go away, without seeming to understand that it would also create problems. In a frank, friendly conversation, the pros and cons of asexuality can certainly be discussed, but some asexual people might feel infantilized if they're perceived as innocent and carefree due to their orientation.

Some non-asexual people have even asked asexual people how to "become asexual," often misunderstanding asexuality as a lack of sex drive. They may perceive their sexual urges as distracting or annoying or as leading them to experience heartache or make bad decisions. But asexual people can't guide anyone on stopping their attraction experiences or changing their sexual desires, and even if they could, it wouldn't necessarily make life easier. The "converted" person would have a different set of problems. Like living with all these misconceptions!

Interestingly, asexual people are often told their lives are so simple, but when they start discussing the intricacies of romantic orientations and types of attraction, they often hear the opposite reaction: "Stop overanalyzing everything! You don't need to make this so complicated!" It's only simple if it's reduced to a sentence. Like any other experience, being asexual has many layers—and it's complex when examined, like any other sexual orientation.

Shouldn't Asexual People Let an Experienced Sexual Partner Change Their Minds?

One of the most frustrating misconceptions about asexuality is the widespread belief that asexual people must not have tried sex—or, similarly, must have tried sex with the wrong partner(s)—and that they can be "converted" through a good sexual encounter. Amazingly, a very high percentage of the people who come up with this one believe themselves to be *just* the one to carry out the experiment! What do asexual people have to lose by "just trying it," right? Can't those stubborn people just open their minds and let someone show them a good time?

Some asexual people *have* tried it. Some asexual people don't want to for the same reason that many heterosexual people don't feel obligated (or even able) to have sex with a member of their own gender to find out if they're really straight. Asexual people don't have to try sex to make sure they wouldn't like it; whether they're attracted to others is the basis of whether they're asexual, and attraction tends to play a big part in most people's choices of who to sleep with. **People usually want sex long before they get it. It's not common for a person to suddenly start finding other people attractive because someone gave them good sex.**

No, sex with a talented partner is not go-

"Even when it's true that the individual in question might like sex if they tried it (in the right circumstances), telling them that they can't know if they're asexual or not if they haven't had sex simply isn't helpful, especially as a response to someone revealing their asexual identity. People should never be made to feel that they need to have sex to feel normal. Ever. If they don't want to have sex, they don't have to have sex. Also, asexuality isn't about not liking sex; it's about not experiencing sexual attraction. People may not be able to know if they like sex or not without trying it, but they can know if they experience sexual attraction or not."
—ANDREW HINDERLITER, *ASEXUAL EXPLORATIONS*

ing to flip a switch for asexual people's ability to become attracted to others. And no, it's not close-minded of asexual people to refuse to "try" a self-proclaimed master of the art. If, for instance, there's a straight guy and his feelings about getting oral sex from a man can't be described as "indifferent," he may understand why he can't expect an asexual person to "just try." Some asexual people aren't only expressing that they aren't excited about or interested in sex; some are actually repulsed by it (as many heterosexual people would be if the only sex available was with their own gender). No one should offer to try it with an asexual person as if it's a favor to them for the benefit of their self-exploration, and no one should act like their unwillingness to have sex is an attitude problem.

Unfortunately, many asexual people feel pressured to go through with it even if they really, really don't want to . . . because they're told over and over again that something worthwhile and fulfilling and beautiful is waiting in coitus, and they're told they "just can't know" until they do it. What if they do try it, still don't experience sexual attraction to others, and realize they were right about themselves in the first place? Do critics nod and finally agree that they did everything reasonable to make sure they were really asexual, and finally start accepting the orientation?

Of course not. Asexual people then hear "If you tried it once and didn't like it, try again! You did it wrong, or with the wrong person! You didn't give it a chance!"

"I didn't enjoy it because I don't enjoy sex with people I'm not attracted to" does not exist to these folks. That just doesn't compute.

Some people who say this are assuming asexual people tried and had a bad experience, which led them to conclude once and for all that sex was not worth it. The first problem with this is that sexual *attraction* is something people usually experience before ever having sex for the first time, and they don't have to prove that they're feeling it or get "switched on" to the idea despite having no inkling that it would feel good. They're compelled by sexual attraction. Asexual people are not. Trying it anyway isn't going to change whether they're attracted to others, though it may help them understand what they're willing to do sexually.

And the second problem with this is that trying "again" still isn't going to satisfy anyone who says this. If an asexual person tries a second time, a third time, a fourth time to like sex and they fail, they will continue to be bombarded with suggestions that they try a different partner, a different gender, a different position, a different time of the month, whatever—as long as they keep trying until they like it. This is absurd because, again, a negative can't be proven.

Lots of people enjoy the idea of making an indifferent or even a gay person realize how great heteronormative sex is, after which, of course, the "converted" will thank the "converter" profusely for the eye-opening, transformative experience. People love thinking that they're so good at sex they could even make an uninterested person crave it. And this, yet again, is a symptom of ego—**this "experiment" would not be for the benefit of the asexual person, but for the purpose of fueling the other person's self-esteem and feelings of accomplishment, as well as confirming their preconceived ideas and narrow perspectives. Again, it's about them, not about the asexual people.**

Asexual people would really rather their experiences be about themselves.

PART FOUR:

IF YOU'RE ASEXUAL (OR THINK YOU MIGHT BE)

Am I Asexual?

A re you sexually attracted to other people? Do you feel the need to make sex a part of your life? Do you have a desire to introduce sexual activities into your relationships? If you answered no to one or more of these questions, you may very well be **asexual**. No expert can "diagnose" you; only you can answer this for yourself.

HOW DO I TELL?

- Do you find other people sexy—in a way that makes you feel sexual desire or arousal, or a way that makes you think sex or sexual touching with that person would be satisfying (regardless of whether you'd actually do it)? If you don't feel this with anyone, you may be **asexual**.
- Do you develop sexual attraction every once in a while, but don't find its pursuit or satisfaction intrinsically rewarding? Some people would call that **asexual**.
- Do you think having sex (or the idea of having sex) is okay, but not very interesting or important? Could you take it or leave it, and find leaving it more convenient or preferable? Some people would call that **asexual**.
- Do you feel sexual attraction sometimes, but only rarely? You may be **gray-sexual**,* and you'll have a lot in common with asexual people if you are.
- Do you sometimes develop sexual attraction when you've already developed other important connections with someone, but never feel sexually attracted to strangers, celebrities, or mere acquaintances? You may be **demisexual**,* and you'll also have a lot in common with asexual people if you are.

* Gray and demi identities are considered to be "on the asexual spectrum"— there are lots of in-betweens! See Part Two of this book for more discussion of romantic identities and types of asexual people, including the gray areas.

Most people have a rather complicated understanding of their situation, and it may be much more nuanced than just yes or no here, but whether a person **experiences sexual attraction** or **finds the word helpful in describing how they feel** is the bedrock answer to whether that person is asexual. It can be pretty difficult to figure out what you're *not* feeling, as opposed to non-asexual people sensing an attraction and recognizing what it must be. Here are some tips:

Educators and activists who address questions on asexuality tend to receive "am I asexual if I . . ." questions consistently, so while the list on the previous page covers the broad strokes, let's take a look at some finer details. None of these are definitive of asexuality, but many of them are common experiences among asexual people. Remember that even if you don't find yourself described here, wondering if you're asexual does suggest that you're having a sexual identity experience outside the norm, and you may find yourself comfortable under the asexual umbrella.

Thinking About Attitudes and Identity:

- Maybe you've wondered if you're the only person in the world to ever not find sex interesting, and you've felt a bit like an alien.
- Maybe you once thought everyone felt how you do about sex, but assumed people were exaggerating their desires when they talked about it.
- Maybe you find people aesthetically appealing, but since it never goes beyond that for you, you don't know what to call yourself.
- Maybe you've realized you're not attracted to cross-sex or cross-gender partners and assumed you must be gay, but have come to find that's not it either.
- Maybe you've mentally dug through all the bad experiences you've had trying to find some reason you aren't able to relate to this "sex thing."
- Maybe you've wondered if you don't know how to love correctly because your love isn't connected to your sexual attraction.
- Maybe it confuses you when people's ultimate fantasies include sex. Your thoughts on getting three wishes, fulfilling a bucket list, or having your last Earthly experiences on Doomsday would not involve sex.

Thinking About Relationships:[1]

- Maybe you would be willing to date, but don't see why everyone else seems so discontent if they're not in a relationship.

---

1 Many of these indicate *aromanticism*, not asexuality, but sometimes aromantic asexual people say their romantic orientation was an early sign of understanding themselves as asexual.

- Maybe you're not interested in dating at all and find it confusing when people ask you how you can stand being chaste or partnerless.
- Maybe you find discussions about romance and dating really tiresome and irrelevant to your life.
- Maybe you'd like to be married, but would rather be more like best friends than have the kind of relationship you see most couples having.
- Maybe you're very romantic and passionate, but just don't find people attractive sexually, and you wonder whether a hopeless romantic like you could still be asexual.
- Maybe you're not sure if you're happy single, but you know it's really frustrating when friends and family pester you to get a partner.
- Maybe you're partnered or even married, and you're having a hard time getting a partner to understand that not desiring them a certain way doesn't mean you don't love them.
- Maybe other people flirt with you and you don't notice, or you say and do things that are interpreted as flirting when you meant nothing of the sort.
- Maybe you have a partner because you are expected to and enjoy being seen as "successful," but don't actually enjoy having a partner intrinsically.

Thinking About Sex:
- Maybe you just don't think about sex and don't understand why it occurs to anyone.
- Maybe you find it harder to understand sexual humor or how sexual motivation works for other people if your mind doesn't go there automatically.
- Maybe it frequently catches you off guard when someone points out another person's sexual appeal, especially if they're saying it about you.
- Maybe people's sexual conversations seem really boring and weird to you, and you don't understand how this holds people's interest for so long.
- Maybe sex itself is intellectually interesting to you, or you find the sociological aspects appealing, but have no desire to participate.
- Maybe it sounds terrible, confusing, and alien to you when people describe sexual desperation: how could they *need* something so badly when you're fine without it?
- Maybe you never dream about sex, or if you do, it's not something that involves you or doesn't seem like a fantasy.

- Maybe appearances of sexual situations in fiction seem random or boring—you may even be inclined to skip the sex scenes.
- Maybe you look at people wearing something that's supposed to be sexy and find yourself distracted by how impractical or bizarre it seems.
- Maybe you like kinky activities but don't want to include sex in your practice.
- Maybe you masturbate and that's all you need or want to do—you have no desire to have this experience with a partner.
- Maybe you masturbate if you feel like it, but don't relate to having an "urge" and could stop anytime if you wanted.
- Maybe you have no desire to masturbate and wouldn't ever try it.
- Maybe you worry that you'll never know how you feel about sex if you don't try it, even though other inexperienced people seem to know they want to.
- Maybe you completely don't relate if friends say someone's sexy, and you've never randomly seen someone and thought "Oh wow, I'd do them."

Engaging in Contact (up to and including sexual contact):
- Maybe you find it off-putting if a partner or potential partner initiates intimate touch.
- Maybe you really enjoy kissing or cuddling and are very sensual, but then don't want it to "escalate."
- Maybe you are willing to have sex, but never find yourself initiating it or suggesting it to partners.
- Maybe you enjoy sex itself but don't feel sexually attracted to a partner and find yourself wondering, "How can I be asexual if I like this?"
- Maybe you have sex or have had sex and found it really underwhelming—even if you enjoyed it, you may have thought, "I can't believe this is what everybody gets so excited about!"
- Maybe you had sex or came close to having sex and found it anxiety-inducing, terrible, gross, unnatural, or very off-putting—and you're further disturbed when people lecture you on how you have to "get over" that to be healthy.
- Maybe you were a lot more intellectually curious than sexually excited about having sex.
- Maybe you have trouble pleasing a partner because you're not into it and don't really know what they would be into, either.
- Maybe you've felt guilty in a relationship and have engaged in physical contact or sex just to avoid hurting the other person or felt ashamed of your lack of interest.

What ties most of these experiences together is that most asexual people have felt like outsiders in this aspect of their lives. Whether this bothers them is highly variable; some asexual people are totally comfortable on the outskirts, while others find it excruciating and devastating, feeling excluded and unable to participate in something so central to most people's lives. That's part of why discovering asexuality and connecting with others can be so liberating, even when it also brings new fears and questions.

Sometimes it's a huge relief to figure out what to call yourself, finally! **But as enlightening as finding a label can be, it isn't absolutely necessary.** You might not want to decide what to call yourself immediately, and that's fine. If you relate to some of what asexual people are talking about, and you don't seem to be feeling sexual interest or attraction the same way your peers do, maybe you should check out some articles, hang out on some forums, and watch some videos to see if you relate. If you find a term that might fit you, feel free to try it out in context and experiment with how you feel about its appropriateness.

But do remember it is not a diagnosis someone else can give to you, and it is not a final decision you can't undo. You can change it if you need to! It's a description. Think of it like your hair color. If you dye your hair, you'll be described differently, right? Change the label you use to fit you. If you turn out to be wrong about being asexual, no harm will have come about from identifying that way when you thought it fit.

If it does fit you, welcome! Asexual communities are very diverse and friendly in many places, and most asexual people have a confusing and frustrating story just like you might. Here's hoping you have a smooth transition into understanding your issues and navigating the world without having to feel inferior or left out or isolated anymore.

But This Changes Everything!

Many asexual people feel a little overwhelmed when they realize they're fundamentally different from most of their friends and family in such an important way. Suddenly, so many assumptions you've made about your life could be wrong! What if everything's going to be an uphill battle for understanding and acceptance from now on?

You'll worry. You may be frustrated and you may doubt yourself and you may wonder how you're supposed to go forward from here. The world has taught you to expect your life to look a certain way, and suddenly nothing is certain anymore. Your relationships are going to be complicated, or maybe you don't want a relationship and you're starting to realize you may never want one, and you don't know what that means for your life. It's not uncommon to go through a period of shock, of depression, even of actual grieving. It's also very common to feel giddy, grateful, relieved, or overcome with a desire to connect with others like yourself. This sounds odd to people who don't see what the big deal is, but for some asexual people who are just realizing their identity, this is world-shaking.

But there are multiple asexual communities and plenty of resources to help you, and many of us have been through what you've been through.

Here are a few reassuring things about asexual people to keep in mind:

REMEMBER:
- Asexuality isn't an illness or a disorder.
- Asexual people can still have relationships if they want them. Asexual people might or might not desire a partner, romantic or otherwise.
- Asexual people have many of the same feelings as everyone else. Non-asexual people eventually realize their asexual friends and family are not that different.
- Asexual people can have many different kinds of romantic orientations.
- Asexual people might or might not like kissing, cuddling, or other intimate touch.
- Asexual people are sometimes told they don't deserve the attention of a significant other if they don't intend to have sex in a relationship, but that's not true for everyone. Every relationship requires communication and compromise.
- Asexual people can be of any gender. Yes, there are asexual men. "All men desire sex, that's just how they are, biologically" is a common misconception.
- Asexual people don't need to accept that they must endure unnecessary therapy or medical tests to "prove" their orientation. Asexuality isn't a diagnosis.
- Asexual people who have suffered abuse, have a mental illness, have a disability or medical condition, take medication, or are autistic are not less asexual. The experience is not less real because of what intersects with it.
- Asexual people might or might not have crushes, get married, and have children.
- Some asexual people engage in self-stimulation, and some others don't.
- Asexual people don't have to be virgins. Having sexual relationships—previously or ongoing—does not invalidate asexuality. Who you sleep with doesn't determine what orientation you are.
- It's possible to enjoy sex itself without feeling sexual attraction to one's partner. Some asexual people are sex-repulsed or sex-neutral, but those who enjoy sex do exist. Sexual attraction is not the same thing as sexual behavior.

Should I Come Out?

This always depends on you. If you were heterosexual, or if you were gay, bisexual, poly-sexual, or pansexual, would you share that with your parents, loved ones, friends, co-work-ers, teachers, online pals, etc.? Most people do feel like sexual orien-

> "Coming out to people and helping educate others on asexuality has given me the confi-dence to insert myself into a sexually driven world. Instead of standing on the outside of it wondering how I fit in, it forces me to carve out a place for myself. When any of us comes out it forces other people to make room for asexuali-ty."
>
> —AUDACIOUS ACE, ASEXUALITY UNABASHED

tation is an important part of their lives, and they feel it's important to include their loved ones in their realization. Some asexual people who come out enjoy a self-affirming experience and believe they're contributing to asexual visibility through disclosing their orientation. However, **it's not necessary to come out if you aren't ready or you aren't comfortable**. As you may have no-ticed based on the other sections in this book, asexual people don't have it easy when it comes to being understood by the majority. You will be misunderstood and you will get flak.

If experiencing pushback or criticism would overwhelm you and you're scared to invite it, don't beat yourself up. Just wait, and if one day you're ready, then come out only to trusted people. If you're worried about how a particular friend or relative will react to the news for *their* sake, you aren't obligated to tell them.

If you don't know how someone will react to asexuality, sometimes you can find opportunities to test them by sending them an article about asexuality and asking what they think or bringing up asexuality as a conversation topic without telling them you identify that way. You may be dismayed that people you care about are as close-minded as they are, but you may also be pleasantly surprised by some people's willingness to listen.

Some asexual folks really want to share their orientation but find it hard to start the conversation. Some good conversation starters that don't seem too awkward might include wearing an asexual-specific shirt or button (some out-right state an asexual message on them, while others might be more subtle like a design of the asexual flag), mentioning an interaction you had on an asexual website, or announcing your orientation during an arranged awareness event; Asexual Awareness Week happens once a year, and you can take advantage of it to come out when loads of resources are available to link to in the media or around the community. If you don't want to schedule a sit-down talk to come out to loved ones, some of these techniques can invite *them* to start the conversation.

> "Occasionally I am jealous of gay people who can sometimes come out relatively tactfully just by mentioning the gender of an ex or a current partner. So I started channeling that feeling productively by thinking about low-key, easy ways to come out while not having to direct the conversation immediately into Asexuality 101 unless I really want it to go there. I often like doing Asexuality 101, but not necessarily when I am trying to socialize and get to know someone better."
>
> —Sciatrix, *Writing From Factor X*

There are some folks in asexual communities who feel it is an asexual person's duty to become a spokesperson since there are so few of us, and that we need every voice. **But honestly, some asexual people just want to be asexual people. That's okay.** It's good to be prepared for the types of questions people throw at you, but sometimes people feel their personal lives are none of anyone's business (especially since the curious tend to ask personal questions with no warning, like *"Do you masturbate?"*—sometimes in group settings or other uncomfortable places). There are ways to avoid attention if you don't want it, and you shouldn't be made to feel like you're a bad person if you don't want to educate every ignorant person.

If you don't want to use the word *asexual* but don't want to pretend to be another sexual orientation either, a line that works well is "I've just never met anyone I'm interested in that way, and I'm fine with that for now." Sometimes well-meaning co-workers or family members can misinterpret singlehood or lack of sexual motivation as loneliness and continue to obliviously push matchmaking requests or questions onto you, and you have the right to ask them to stop this without making up an excuse. Some asexual people have combated this problem by wearing a fake wedding wing, making up a fake partner, or claiming to be another sexual orientation to help reject advances. Truth or truth by omission is best if possible, but if you feel *safer* with lies that protect you from violent or triggering experiences, you shouldn't have to feel awful about using them.

How Should I Handle the Criticism?

One roadblock to coming out for some asexual people is the fear of rejection and combative questions. This is a very real concern, because almost invariably, it happens with at least some of the people you come out to. Depending on whom you're disclosing to and what the context is, you may be asked explicit questions about how your genitals work. You may be encouraged to try sex toys. You may be prodded for your romantic history, laughed at while people suggest you were abused or molested, mockingly assigned a homosexual identity either as if it's an insult or as if it's something you need to admit to yourself, and condescended to by "concerned" people who want you to see a doctor even if they have no history of caring about your health otherwise. It's not easy.

If the above suggestions sound appalling, that's because they are. And why should you have to deal with such things? You don't! **If a question you are asked is too personal, you have the right act as revolted as you feel.** There is no excuse for someone to ask for intricate and intimate details about your anatomy, your sex life, your masturbatory habits, or your possible trauma. Be really firm about it if this happens to you and you don't find it appropriate— make it clear that questions like that are really offensive.

Sometimes sarcasm works: "Okay, you just met me and you're asking me about my vagina. That's really classy." Or point blank reasoning: "If I wasn't asexual, would you think it was okay to ask me questions about dildos?" And *especially* if they demand details of whether you've had an abusive experience— regardless of whether you have—feel free to tell them what a hideously inappropriate question that is.

If you're uncomfortable dealing with these sorts of queries, pawn people off on other resources (this book, for instance!) or give *general* answers to specific questions. This helps a lot. If someone asks you if

"Generally straightforward works best. 'Just so you know, I'm asexual.' Hey, that wasn't too bad! If you don't make a big deal out of it—and don't give any impression that you're looking for approval—people will be less likely to give you trouble for it."
—QUEENIE, *CONCEPT AWESOME*

you masturbate and you don't want to avoid the question but don't feel comfortable discussing it, tell them, "Some asexual people do, some don't. Asexuality isn't about behavior. It's about attraction." If someone wants to know whether **your** parts work, tell them, "Most asexual people do have the ability to become aroused. Being asexual doesn't mean having nonfunctional genitals. But they're not attracted to people any more than someone who gets an erection at the proctologist is attracted to the doctor's finger." Deflect.

Unfortunately, sometimes the people who corner you and interrogate you are your family, your loved ones, your partner(s), or your long-time friends. These people theoretically *do* have a history with you, which would suggest intimate questions are fair game, and you may not know what to do if a concerned parent or protective best friend decides asexuality is a disorder and intends to talk you out of it. This process can sometimes be demeaning and scary, so if you have concerned loved ones who think they're just trying to help you, please remember the following things that might help put their worry into perspective:

- They may be concerned about your health and may believe every healthy person feels sexual attraction and has a desire to find partners.
- They may believe asexuality is a decision they can convince you to give up.
- They may think there's no solution that doesn't involve *you* changing.
- They may think you owe their perspective a try, but that the reverse isn't applicable.
- They may think you'll be sad without a romantic partner, a sexual partner, marriage, and/or children (or know they would be), and believe you cannot/will not have these relationships and experiences if you are asexual.
- They may really believe they will be *helping* you by "fixing" this.

So, remember—we might roll our eyes and figure they're just being obnoxious with all this concern trolling,[2] but **normally this sort of "intervention" from close friends or family really is fueled by (admittedly misguided) concern for you**. They may think you're condemning yourself to a life of loneliness. They may think this is a decision you're making out of desperation, or they may think you're confused and crying for help. They may have little ability to empathize and really can't conceive of a person being both single and happy (if you don't desire a partner), both abstinent and well-adjusted (if you're not interested in sex), or completely satisfied without feeling sexual attraction (regardless of what you do with partners). So before you treat any "concerned conversation" as an attack, please do take these perspectives into consideration. It's very likely they just want to help you, and your job at that point is to make sure they understand where their "help" is appropriate and where it is not.

But what if you're getting the third degree and getting backed into a corner? What should you do? Always try respectful responses first, but don't be afraid of being confrontational if it's warranted. If detractors insult you, reframe

---

2 *Concern trolling* is a slang phrase that refers to a method of undermining a position or perspective by pretending to care about the well-being of the person holding said position or perspective. People who concern-troll asexual people may claim they're worried about the asexual person's health or happiness, for example, but everything they say is geared toward discrediting asexuality as an orientation.

something about your life in an unflattering way and/or lie about it, make unrealistic or shame-based predictions, accuse you of anything they shouldn't, or try to bargain with you about your obligations regarding dating or sex, you can feel free to either treat them like they're ridiculous or end the conversation.

You deserve respect and you shouldn't be made to feel like you're on the defensive when you're talking about asexuality. You shouldn't have to prove how you feel, feel as though your critic is automatically right if you can't express yourself effectively, or feel that their education is your responsibility.

Here are some tips.

If your conversation partner is employing fairly RESPECTFUL conversational decorum, try the following techniques and phrases:

- Get the conversation partner alone. It's much harder to "fight" a group of people who are all head-nodding and throwing out protests that you're expected to defend. This isn't always possible, but it's especially effective with a person who has brought this up with you more than once.
- Start the conversation yourself (with a person who has historically had issues with the topic or with someone you're coming out to). Come to the discussion prepared, and take advantage of the fact that the other person may not have done a lot of thinking about it while you have.
- Point out that you aren't alone in being asexual. Sometimes people back down when they find out there are whole asexual communities, with research, articles, interviews, and documentaries on the subject. If you're not just an oddball who supposedly "doesn't want to have sex," sometimes they start feeling less like you need to defend your orientation and more like *they* would need to defend not being knowledgeable about its existence.
- Give them information. This sometimes works even in combative situations; send a link, hand them a pamphlet or a URL reference, give them a phrase to search online or an article title to read later, quote a video, mention an asexual community, tell them to watch the documentary *(A)sexual*. If they resist looking at your material, **ask them why they are not willing to educate themselves if they still expect you to listen to their objections.**
- Accept their criticism and listen. Let them talk, and let them finish sentences. And then follow up with "I understand why you might say that, *but*. . . ." Explain where they're confused, mixing up terms, making

assumptions, exaggerating, or misinterpreting. But be willing to nod and hear their concerns.

- Remind them that you didn't "decide" to be asexual, and that this isn't something they can talk you out of through reasoning. You're using it as a description for how you feel and will continue to identify with the label until or unless it does not fit you. Some detractors relax when you say that it's possible you'll change in the future, but stress that you're not admitting it's likely. "Never" looks the same as "not yet" when we're still in the present.

- Ask *them* questions. Asexuality discussions are usually full of demands for the asexual people to justify their orientation. Turn it around by asking them questions such as "Why do you think asexuality can't exist?" or "Do you understand what it means?" Getting them on the defensive sometimes makes them put their possibly incorrect conceptions into words so you can correct them.

- Ask them to ask you questions. Be open to answering them and take ownership of the conversation. This way you will feel less like you're being badgered and cornered; you're inviting their curiosity and making this a voluntary procedure.

- Ask for respect. If necessary, *remind* them to be respectful. If they ask a question that is nasty or too personal or deliberately derailing the conversation, remind them that you're capable of describing your own feelings and you expect to be talked to politely. Most people don't want to disrespect you and will pull back if you suggest they're being disrespectful.

- Refer them to an authority who takes questions if you're sick of it. There are many asexual Q&A resource bloggers who have a lot of patience and will be willing to take the heat off you if you need it.

Now, if your conversation is heated, combative, offensive, full of confrontation, deliberately abusive, or may include yelling, try these tips. These people are marginalizing you and telling you that you aren't feeling what you're feeling, and you have the right to use strong measures in teaching them that isn't okay.

If your conversation partner is employing DISRESPECTFUL or ABUSIVE behavior, try the following techniques and phrases:

- Express personal disappointment in the other person's refusal to respect you. Abject nastiness is usually unnecessary, but sometimes you can goad people into listening to you. Try "You really hate learning anything new, huh?" or "Have you ever thought about taking a class on better communication skills? Listening obviously isn't your strong suit." If they're not going to be open to your perspective, why should you be open to theirs? Reminding them of this sometimes allows you to guide the conversation back to the more civil techniques.

- Demand to know why they're so obsessed with *your* sex life. This works especially well if you're being harassed in a group setting and the ringleader has put you on the spot on purpose. Shooting back with "This person is really obsessed with my sex life" sometimes gets people off your back. And sometimes suggesting the person is digging so hard because of being sexually interested in you puts them on the defensive.

- Question their motivation and their need to invalidate you. "Is this *really* about me, or do you just have a hard time getting your head around it?" Ask if they get off on condemning you. Ask if they feel it's easier to be ignorant. If someone else cares so much more about your sex life than you do, sometimes making them feel like their attention is inappropriate will make them stop.

- If they're concern trolling, ask them if they need printouts of your fitness routines and food intake. Obviously if they're so concerned about your *health*, they should want the whole picture, right? Oh, but somehow only your sexuality is of interest? What's really going on here?

- Push them into having an even discussion with you by asking if they're even listening. Imply that you are at a lecture. Act disappointed that they apparently can't be bothered to listen to you since they're so intent on talking *at* you. Ask them to agree to let you speak uninterrupted for a certain amount of time, and scold them if they interrupt.

- When they start hammering you with the same old objections that have been voiced a hundred times, point out how common they are or say "Oh, a lot of people make that mistake." Better yet, bring up others they haven't hit yet. Usually people of this description think their objections are really original, and they hate being reminded that we've heard them before. When they ask whether you're sure you're not gay or if you just had bad sex, respond, "Oh, you missed a few. Aren't you going to ask me if I got my hormones checked or whether I was abused as a child? Usually those two come before the 'are you gay?' question." This helps point out that we've thought of these things before and didn't just wake up one day "deciding not to have sex."

- If you're dealing with heterosexual folks who think a virgin asexual person needs to "just try it," ask if they would be willing to "try" being gay. Ask them why you're held to different standards than they are—why you're expected to try sex you know you don't want, while they can just know they're not gay without trying any kind of sex they don't desire. This usually doesn't work with bisexual or gay people because many of them can imagine going through with such things (and may have actually done so), but since heterosexual people are the ones who typically have the most rigid views on sexuality and how it "should" be, this is a good piece of ammunition.

- Turn nasty questions around. If they ask whether you're subscribing to an Internet fad, ask them whether they got the idea to have sex from porn on the Internet. If they ask what traumatic event happened to you to make you asexual, ask them, "Did something *happen* to you to make you so threatened by people who don't want you?" If they tell you you've just never been with the right person, say, "I'm sure we could turn you straight if we just hooked you up with a really cute girl." (Altered as appropriate, of course.) Oh, and if a straight person has actually tried same-gender sex and supposedly determined they're definitely straight, ask them why having sex is supposed to "cure" your asexuality if same-gender sex didn't "cure" their straightness or accuse them of needing to try multiple part-ners before they're "sure," just like people say you need to try it a bunch of times with multiple people before anyone will believe you're asexual.
- If they start recycling points, tell them you already rebutted those and end the conversation. This isn't an opportunity for them to just tune you out until it's their turn to talk.

You never know what item will work to turn a critic into an ally. Sometimes it just takes the right point and the wheels will start turning. They will realize they were being ignorant, abusive, or dismissive, ultimately helping to make the world harder for a largely invisible population. Most people don't want to be that jerk. You can take the lead on helping them get there, but unfortunately, some people have to be cajoled into even giving you a chance to talk. Beliefs about sexuality are so ingrained in our society and so established in some people's minds that challenging those assumptions can sometimes bring a massive fight.

You might be pleasantly surprised by who finds asexuality easy to grasp, and sorely disappointed by who refuses to support you. In some cases, you may find that you just plain can't get through to someone, and your relationship with them may become strained or intolerable because of it. When a person is con-stantly invalidating you or subjecting you to mocking or regular harassment over your orientation, sometimes it's best to distance yourself from that person if it's possible or talk to other people in that person's life and ask them to assist you in avoiding the subject (or avoiding interaction completely).

It's not absolutely necessary that you find a way to get through to every person; educating them is not your responsibility if you've decided it's just too stressful or emotionally exhausting or pointless. **You may try coming out to people you don't know well first, if you feel that's appropriate, just to get a taste for the kinds of things people will be asking and a little experience saying the words out loud.**

If you're not comfortable with face-to-face interaction or you're not a good speaker, write the necessary parties a letter. You can even include a pamphlet (for hard-copy letters) or links to resources (for electronic communication) if you feel more confident with backup.

And read some coming-out stories on asexual communities and blogs around the Internet! You might feel compelled to share some of your own experiences or just feel more confident knowing other people have been through the same things and come out—ha—on the other side.

What If I'm a Teenager? Everyone Keeps Calling Me a "Late Bloomer."

As mentioned elsewhere in this book, most people begin to figure out their sexual identity during their teenage years, so while the majority of teens are forming their first sexual interests and relationships, asexual teens will be realizing there's something different about how they relate to their peers. And when they look for help from adults they trust, asexual teens often face condescension and disbelief because some older people may react to asexuality as if it is a phase, fake, case of late blooming, or lack of self-awareness.

When coming out, asexual teens will often be told (especially by parents or other adults) they are too young to know what they want. This isn't true. Yes, it's true that sexual orientation is fluid for some people. And it's possible

> "People are told 'You're just a late bloomer.' People are told 'Wait. Sexuality will emerge.' Yet these hearers ask themselves how long must they wait to 'know' they're not a late bloomer. Till they're sixteen? Till they're twenty-six? Till they're sixty-two? Must life be spent in perpetual waiting to eventually 'bloom' into being sexual?"
>
> —ANDREW HINDERLITER, *ASEXUAL EXPLORATIONS*

you'll identify as something else later in your life if you happen to be fluid or you have experiences that make you want to change how you describe yourself. But for you, *asexual* is the term you're using now because you aren't experiencing the same attractions everyone else seems to, and it seems the best fit for now.

"I've never found anyone attractive that way, so I'll identify as asexual unless that changes for me" works for some younger folks trying to explain it to older adults. After all, past and present are the best predictors we have of the future. Your maturity and self-awareness may be more readily accepted and respected if you acknowledge that you do not know the future. (And neither do they.) However, arguing with older people about this is sometimes futile; some of them will not believe you. If they claim you're just going through a phase or that you will find your "real" sexuality when you're more mature, they're unlikely to be sympathetic or listen to you. You'll probably have another disappointing or condescending experience if you get confrontational about your maturity because they already think you aren't mature enough to truly know yourself if they say this.

Some older people react poorly to a young asexual person coming out because they're convinced it's a declaration against sex—that you're all about swearing off sex forever. Sometimes you can get a better response if you reassure your older friends and loved ones that asexuality is a description, not a decision.

If someone in your life has a history of dismissing your opinion or your wisdom because of your age, you may either come prepared for this or simply make the decision not to come out to those people at this point in your life. Coming out isn't a necessity, and if you feel safer and happier without labeling yourself outwardly, you can always wait until you're more likely to be respected or choose to avoid labeling yourself to these people indefinitely.

Asexual teens certainly do have the capacity to understand themselves. If you are in your teens and think you might be asexual, take heart. Many of us who identify as asexual later in life knew it when we were teens, too. If you find yourself lost as to how to explain yourself or just want to talk to others who understand, there is an extensive list of forums and helpful websites in the Resources section of this book.

What If I'm Already in a Relationship, or Want to Be? What Do I Tell My Partner(s)?

Some asexual people find it more satisfying and simpler to choose only other asexual partners for their significant others, and this is one possible way to go about becoming and staying partnered. But—for reasons discussed more extensively in Part Two on Asexual Relationships—finding a compatible asexual/

asexual relationship is rare. Asexual social networking sites (mentioned in the Part Six, the Resources section) can help find others if this is the route you choose, but it's much more likely that partner-desiring people will find themselves trying to negotiate relationships with non-asexual partners.

Dealing with your partner(s) as an asexual person is a special issue, especially if you only discover you're asexual after you've been dating a long time or are already married to someone who is not asexual. Most people do assume that sex is an expected part of a romantic partnership and tend to believe something is wrong if you don't want them that way.

You may have already experienced some hiccups in your relationship because of this. You may feel pressured. You may have had sex you did not desire because you were taught it was expected. You may have wondered why you didn't feel enthusiastic about sex the way your partner(s) might be. You may have been confronted about your failure to initiate or vocally enjoy sex. Your partner(s) may have expressed feeling hurt by your refusal of sex or lack of excitement over it. But if you've realized you're asexual and that's what's behind all the mismatched desires in your relationship, you can now do something about it. It is no longer something you must accept as being "wrong with you" for not wanting what they want, just like nothing is wrong with *them* for wanting more sex than you do.

The most important elements of making relationships work are compromise and communication. "Compromise" does not mean you, as the asexual person, necessarily need to be the only one doing the compromising. You probably already know—and have experienced firsthand—the attitude many people hold regarding sexual relations within a relationship (especially a marriage), but **no one is obligated to ever have sex with anyone for any reason**, and if you have been taught that it's the only way to show your full love for another person, this will take some time to unlearn. People show their love in many different ways, and you can focus on and eventually internalize the acts of love that are authentic for you.

Someone whose love for you is contingent upon your sexual activity with them is being abusive if they try to guilt or force you into giving them sex you don't want to give. They should be able to acknowledge that people show love in different ways and not brand you as "not loving them enough" if sex isn't how you'd choose to show it. They may truly love you, but you don't have to put up with abuse to be loved.

You may be being manipulated or shamed if you hear phrases like "I guess you don't really love me completely" or "I do a lot for you and you can't just do this little thing for me?" or "If this keeps up, I'm going to have to get it from somewhere else, you know." If a partner tries to guilt you into sex or treat you like you're unreasonable for not engaging in it, you will need to have a serious talk about communication or you will need to think seriously about going your separate ways because no one has the right to demand sex from you. If you wonder whether your situation is abusive, additional resources can help answer that question.[3] If you ever find yourself in crisis because of a partner's abuse—whether threatened or carried out—domestic violence hotlines[4] can coach you on immediate safety and steps to protect yourself.

Most partners, friends, concerned loved ones, and therapists will approach a partnership like yours by trying to "fix" an asexual partner. "How can we make asexual partners deal with sex more?" they might wonder. "How can we fix the situation so non-asexual partners get the sex they need and everyone will be happy?" Notice the blame gets placed on the asexual partner(s). That's not fair. Everyone in the relationship should bear an equal amount of responsibility for its peace and happiness. First, try to encourage everyone involved—especially your partner(s)—to understand that you have a *mismatch of sexual needs*, not a situation that is one person's fault for wanting sex too much or not enough.

If you are in a relationship and you have come out to your partner(s), you should try to be understanding at first if they are upset by it. Let them be upset, try to be reassuring, and tell them you'll try to figure out together how everyone involved can be happy during the next conversation. If they seem understanding, though, and want to figure out how to negotiate right away, one great thing to do is have each of you figure out your must-haves, your dealbreakers, and what you're willing to compromise. Talk it over informally, create a list based on your own experiences and desires, or use a template from a relationship negotiation resource.[5]

You will need to examine how you truly feel about sex. If you know you don't desire it but can enjoy it from time to time or just enjoy what it means for you and your partner(s) to be together, you may want to list "occasional sex" or "regular sex" as a compromise for you. However, if you're completely opposed to sex and do not want to have it ever (or ever again), you can consider "must have at least occasional sex" a dealbreaker. Consider what kinds of sex and what kinds of

3 One helpful website to use in diagnosing abusive relationships is *Love Is Respect* (www.loveisrespect.org). Users can take quizzes, look up information about types of abuse, and access resources.
4 In the United States, the National Domestic Violence Hotline provides confidential counseling and advice through their toll-free telephone line—(800) 799-7233—or their website at www.thehotline.org. The website also has a chat feature and lists of local organizations that can help. For help outside the United States, a list of resources is provided by the National Coalition Against Domestic Violence at www.ncadv.org/resources/InternationalOrganizationResources.php.
5 Checklists can be used or modified from the resources at *Scarleteen* (www.scarleteen.com/article/advice/yes_no_maybe_so_a_sexual_inventory_stocklist) or *SmartHotFun* (smarthotfun.com/wantwillwontchart).

physical intimacy you like or will allow, what you're willing to do, and what you do *not* want to do. Will you still engage in kissing? Necking? Petting? Foreplay? Cuddling? BDSM? Toys? Fetishes? Sensual massage? Sleeping in the same bed?

Also consider compromises you can make in your relationship: Are you willing to continue or begin an open relationship? Polyamory, non-monogamy?[6] Are you open to sex toys, or non-penetrative forms of sex, or manual stimulation, or mutual masturbation, or watching a partner use a toy? Would any of that satisfy your partner(s) while not requiring your own lines to be crossed? Would the non-asexual partner(s) prefer to privately self-stimulate or go without sex rather than pursue alternate avenues? Some non-asexual people like sex but don't require it, and that has to be their call. They may feel that the positive experiences you've built together unrelated to sex are too important to lose over an incompatibility of your sex drives, sexual attraction, or sexual willingness.

It's not very common for a non-asexual person to give up all sex for a relationship with a sex-repulsed asexual partner, but it can happen and has happened. Honesty must be stressed, though, because a non-asexual person saying "I'll just go without sex and take care of my urges myself" is sometimes harder than the person anticipates, and it could possibly lead to undiscussed affairs, frustration, or bitterness. If you're an asexual person and a non-asexual partner volunteers to just cut off sex with no substitute or compromise, be sure to follow up later with the partner and discuss their satisfaction and happiness, leaving room for renegotiation. They should also do that with you and let you feel comfortable approaching them if something you've agreed to try is making you unhappy. Discussions should primarily focus on how *you* feel ("I feel we don't focus on intimacy unless we're having sex") rather than *their* actions ("You don't give me intimate attention unless you're going to get sex"); this keeps the conversations from becoming accusatory or hostile.

As you can see, there are many sexual and intimate compromises a partnership can negotiate, and not all of them require the asexual partner(s) to begin or continue with sex they may not want, nor do they all require the non-asexual partner(s) to go without. Do keep in mind, however, that some non-asexual people will feel betrayed if they find out you were never attracted to them the way they thought you were—since they assumed you would not have been having sex or a relationship with them if you weren't—and they may no longer *want* to be intimate with you if you just aren't into it like they are. Many asexual people

6 A good asexual-friendly resource for those who might want to learn about approaching polyamory is Franklin Veaux's website *More Than Two*: www.morethantwo.com.

just didn't know their feelings weren't the norm, may have been ashamed of their disinterest, or may have felt it was unacceptable to bring it up, so if this comes up, do stress that it wasn't an intentional manipulation.

It's okay if one of *their* dealbreakers is you not being sexually attracted to them. If they absolutely cannot deal with that, or if they require sex in their relationships and you are not willing to engage in it, it's okay if you agree to dissolve the relationship. (Easier said than done if it's a long-term relationship and/or a marriage, but not all partnerships can negotiate compatibility, and it's better to call it quits than to have any partner constantly frustrate or abuse another partner for the sake of staying together.)

Keep in mind that no matter what anyone says—especially if it's in the heat of a bad breakup—asexual people are *not* completely incompatible in relationships with non-asexual people. "That kind of relationship just can't work, *period*" is a misleading and ultimately untrue thing to say, and anyone who says it is speaking for people who aren't them, so don't believe it if anyone tries to convince you that your love life will be hopeless unless you partner with another asexual person. Everyone is different. You may just need to be better prepared to enter the relationship fully aware of what you're bringing to the table and what you're willing to compromise on.

If you do decide to go to relationship therapy or sex therapy, partners should be aware that not all professionals in the field accept the validity of asexuality. They may end up doing what so many other people do: focus on the asexual partner(s) as the problem. If your therapy simply tries to make you accept or initiate sex more often to satisfy a more eager partner, you should call them out on it, because **coercing someone into unwanted sex and telling them they should like it is abuse**. Unless you have willingly entered therapy specifically trying to increase your sexual enjoyment, appetite, or aptitude, it is wrong for them to focus entirely on changing you but not your non-asexual partner(s), and you should go to a different professional who believes your input is just as important.

So Where Do I Go From Here?

If you've realized you're asexual and you want to know what's next besides coming out and working on your relationships, you may be craving understanding and community. It is strongly recommended that, if you want to share your story, get coming-out advice from real people, find asexual friends, or learn more about asexuality in general, you should join an asexuality-based online community. Many asexual people experience relief and joy from finally getting to meet others who have been through what they've been through. A list of communities is available in Part Six.

Some LGBTQ groups are asexual-inclusive, so if you feel comfortable joining a queer community in your area, you can find out whether they already welcome people of your orientation or whether they'd like to include you and have you bring an asexual perspective. (Asexuality is generally unquestioned in these groups if you are *also* another queer identity, like if you're romantically attracted to same-gender partners or are transgender. If you're heteroromantic or aromantic and you're cisgender, though, some groups may not want to welcome you unless it's as an ally.)

Asexual-specific meetup groups are becoming more popular now, too, and events are often arranged through asexuality.org or meetup services. There are even asexual dating sites if you're looking for someone of your orientation to partner with. Read some of the "I've discovered I'm asexual" stories in the forums and blogs around the Internet, and you may be surprised how similar everyone's story sounds. Ask some questions[7]—anonymously if you need to—and compare your experiences with others'. And though some people don't feel comfortable in online communities or find them too problematic or confusing to be helpful, they can still sometimes be used to find organizations or other individuals to meet with offline.

Hopefully it won't be long before you feel at home and accepted, inside and out.

---

7 Try *Asexual Advice*, a blog that takes submissions either through Tumblr accounts or anonymously: asexualadvice.tumblr.com.

PART FIVE:
IF SOMEONE YOU KNOW IS ASEXUAL
(OR MIGHT BE)

A Message for Non-Asexual People

First of all: thank you very much for picking up this book.

The best thing you can do for asexual people is to try to understand **what** we are in macro and **who** we are in micro. And even if you're not looking for this information because of a personal connection with an asexual person in your life, you will be helping to make the world less hostile and more welcoming for all of us by becoming more aware of our issues and experiences.

We really appreciate your willingness to try to understand us, and hopefully this book will make that journey as easy as possible.

What Does It All Mean?

So maybe someone you love or know just came out to you as asexual, and maybe you're concerned. Maybe you're curious. Maybe you're happy for them or proud of them. Maybe you're worried that something's wrong with the person, you want to know more about how the person thinks, you're sad that they might not have a great relationship or children because of it, or you hope there's a cure.

If someone you know is asexual and you want to talk about it, keep these two pieces of advice in mind: One, do more listening than talking/asking when it comes to the asexual person's perspective. Two, educate yourself on the subject; a list of helpful resources is included in the last chapter of this book. You may be surprised how much the asexual people in your life might appreciate you taking the initiative to learn about it. Your asexual loved ones don't have to be the main source of all your information on asexuality, though if they say something about their own experience that contradicts your research, you shouldn't use it to invalidate them.

This book's other sections cover what asexuality is, what asexual people's lives are like, and what misconceptions they face. However, here's a quick cheat sheet of that material if you came straight to this chapter first:

Asexuality is: An orientation describing people who don't feel sexually attracted to anyone. (It's not a behavior, like abstinence. It's an orientation, like gay, straight, or bi.)

Asexuality is not: It's not a sickness or a mental illness. It's not the same thing as celibacy. It's not proof that someone has been abused. It is not "caused" by a medical issue or negative experience. It's not a hurdle people should be expected to "get over." It's not the same thing as having a low sex drive. It doesn't refer to a person who is a virgin or vows never to have sex. It doesn't refer to a person who has had bad sex and sworn off it. It isn't about hating people who have sex, hating other people in general, or failing to meet the right person. It isn't hidden homosexuality. It isn't a religious statement. It isn't just a phase. It isn't a diagnosis or a cry for attention or a reason to seek therapy. It doesn't mean a person is ugly or socially awkward or lonely.

It might surprise you: That asexual people can have romantic relationships and marriages if they want to. That asexual people may negotiate sexual relationships if they want to. That some asexual people want to be parents. That some asexual people feel other (nonsexual) types of attraction. That some asexual people masturbate. That scientific studies have been done to examine asexuality as a sexual orientation. That asexual people can be any gender, sex, race, religion, or national origin. That asexual people can experience prejudice and discrimination for their orientation. That people can have disabilities / have mental or physical illnesses / take medication / be abuse survivors / be autistic **and** be asexual without these intersections "causing" each other or delegitimizing any of their realities. That most asexual people don't want to be "cured."

If you only have *more* questions now and you want to know more about something covered above, before asking the asexual person in your life for your own individual education session, consider reading the rest of this book—including the section aimed at asexual people (Part Four) and the "resources" section (Part Six) with references to articles, scientific research, and personal perspectives. Some of your questions may be answered without unnecessary awkwardness, especially if you have some very personal questions about masturbation, sexuality, sexual experimentation, gender, medical issues, or abuse history. Some of the natural questions you have might upset the asexual person for reasons you may not understand at this point, and a little preemptive research can help you avoid losing the asexual person's trust while you try to figure out what asexuality means for the asexual people in your life.

This section will assume that you want to support asexual people—that you'd like to be an ally. **The asexual population very much needs people like you, and we do want you to understand us.** However, we do understand that some people who read about us might be hoping or believing that asexuality is a phase or a curable disease and might not be willing to accept it as an orientation. Regardless of your reasons for opening this book, hopefully you'll be open to hearing some advice on how to foster a positive discussion about asexuality. Especially if you are very close to an asexual person, your reaction may be of utmost importance.

What Do Asexual People Want? How Can I Make Them Feel Accepted?

The single most common and resoundingly consistent answer from asexual communities is that we want you to acknowledge that asexuality exists.

Maybe this sounds easy, but keep in mind asexual people are a largely unknown population. The discrimination they face isn't particularly visible; they're rarely oppressed through deliberate action, but they *are* living every day with little to no acknowledgment of a central aspect of their lives. And yes, *that still constitutes living in a prejudicial environment*, though no one is comparing it with more violent expressions of oppression or suggesting we have it as bad or worse. (In other words, we sometimes hear comments like "but other minorities have much bigger problems." Those aren't helpful statements because we aren't trying to figure out who has it worse and only focus on the problems of the most disadvantaged groups.)

We're saying that it means the world to asexual people if we're included when sexual orientations are examined and that we want to be understood as just one more acceptable way to be.

So How Can I Acknowledge Their Existence?

Obviously it'd seem a little silly if an asexual person mentioned being asexual and you jumped in with "Oh, hi there. I believe you exist!" So how can you show that you acknowledge their existence?

First, you should be careful with your blanket statements about sexuality, especially when it comes to comparing lack of sexual interest with lack of personhood, or suggesting that "everybody" needs sex or is driven by sex. You can make sure the orientation gets represented in academic discussions or surveys of sexuality if you are involved in the creation or distribution of these materials.

You can refrain from assuming everyone who's single is trying to be otherwise (since plenty of people, including some asexual people, don't want partners), and if an asexual person brings up the subject, just offer acceptance in your own way. **You can approach people in general without assuming everyone feels sexual attraction until proven otherwise.**

Ultimately, if you take care *not* to assume everyone you meet experiences sexual attraction or is interested in sex, and you remain mindful of including asexual people even outside of their presence, you'll be helping to bring asexuality's existence into the common consciousness.

How you support the asexual people in your life is going to vary widely depending on what your relationship with them is like. But in general, if an asexual person is coming out and wants you to be partial to this revelation, the best thing you can do is *listen.*

> "Right now, coming out entails playing educator, representative of my sexuality, and terrified person trying to share something important all at the same time. (I try not to show I'm terrified.) Have I ever mentioned that it is difficult to play educator when you've just bared a secret, important part of yourself and you know that total confusion is one of the best-case scenarios?"
> —SCIATRIX, *WRITING FROM FACTOR X*

This person is expressing trust toward you, and even if you have some misgivings about asexuality or don't understand what it means in this particular asexual person's case, if you don't listen and at least try to process what is being said, anything you say against it during this delicate time may cause a shutdown or a withdrawal. The asexual person may regret being honest with you and may be completely closed to discussion with you on this topic if you don't keep your mind open. Let us speak, and consider what we say without automatic condemnation. That's all we can ask.

And you can't go wrong with telling us you support us and care for us, establishing an accepting attitude before asking any questions.

Now, if you have a friend or family member whom *you* think might be asexual but they have *not* discussed it with you, you may be in a different situation. Are you trying to find out whether someone you know is asexual? Or maybe someone you know is confused about their identity and is dropping hints about their attraction experiences that make you think perhaps they are asexual but haven't heard of the orientation? There are a couple ways you can approach this situation if *you* are the one who wants to bring it up with *them.*

I recommend against specifically asking the person "are you asexual?" or telling them they're probably asexual unless they're asking you explicitly for suggestions on what they might be. If you're hoping to help an asexual person discover what might be their identity, you'll want to bring up the orientation without putting pressure on them to confirm or deny its application to themselves. The best way to casually introduce the topic is to mention or share an article or video or news piece you've seen and express support. Say you think it's great that asexual people are finding a voice or that you are firmly in the "whatever floats your boat" camp. Allying yourself with asexual visibility may help asexual-identified people realize they can trust you and may help asexual people who don't know about the orientation figure out some aspects of their identity that may have been causing them anxiety. You may actually be able to help asexual people find their place in the community by learning more about it yourself.

Is There Anything I Should Avoid Saying or Doing?

Here are some comments we sometimes hear from people who want to be supportive but don't realize what they're saying. (If you'd like a more comprehensive understanding of some of the comments people make to invalidate asexual people, those are discussed in more detail in Part Three of this book.) You may not have even thought of any of these objections, but we do hear them, so I'm going to share why these statements might put us off.

Don't suggest asexuality is actually repressed homosexuality, suppressed trauma, or a disorder. Yes, these things exist and they also can cause lack of interest in pursuing sex, but we don't feel that asexuality is a last resort diagnosis that can only be applied if we've proved it's not anything else.

Don't immediately start trying to be sympathetic by saying you are "sometimes asexual" or that you wish you were; don't suggest you understand completely because you have a low sex drive; and don't list the "bright sides" of our situation. We're probably not asking you to comfort us. Though sometimes it's interesting to discuss it with

> "You think it's easy to be asexual in a world where sex is valued above anything else? You think there's such a thing as an 'asexual media'? Look around you. Most people don't even know asexuality exists. I get told by many people who don't know me that I must be sick, or frigid, or afraid. (. . .) In case you didn't get the message earlier: in no way is it easy being part of a minority sexuality."
> —Jo Qualmann, *A Life Unexamined*

people who once thought they were asexual and turned out not to be. (That's a different discussion.)

There are some things about being asexual that make life easier for some, but "I wish I was like you!" or "you're so lucky!" can come off as infantilizing or condescending—they may think you're saying you're wiser and more mature because of your complicated desires, while their life is probably carefree and easy like that of a child. (Clearly not everyone who says this is implying that their lives are harder, but if you wish to be an ally, you should know you might be interpreted that way if you use that phrasing.)

Incidentally, most of the people who say they "wish they were asexual" are actually expressing that their sexual urges are distracting or annoying. That's a very different thing from "I wish I wasn't attracted to anybody," and **even if you mean well, saying you wish you were a marginalized person does have a partial effect of trivializing what asexual people go through.** Some of us have at times wished we were like you too, but neither of us actually knows what we're asking for if we say so. Probably best to leave it out of a first conversation at least, until you know more about the asexual person's experiences and attitudes.

Don't make assumptions about what our asexuality means, even if the statements technically express support (e.g., "I think it's *great* that you're saving yourself!" or "You must be so spiritually enlightened!").

Don't express that we're selfish or otherwise inferior because you think we will not have children. If you express that your asexual friend or family member is hurting you somehow by acknowledging an orientation that you perceive to result in childlessness, you may make the person feel like their primary worth to you is their offspring. Coming out as asexual is about them. If you are concerned about them having children, especially if you are their parent or grandparent, you should only discuss their reproductive plans in a nurturing way and do not treat them like a disappointment or yourself like a victim. They really aren't trying to hurt you by being asexual, and furthermore, asexual people have certainly been known to have children; if they are so inclined and able, it's still completely possible, either biologically or through adoption.

Don't ask why the asexual person "decided to be asexual," and **don't** ask us to "try" being something else. Much like LGBTQ folks, we commonly hear our identity being understood as a decision. We're often asked to pursue therapy to make sure nothing's wrong with us before we call ourselves asexual. We're regularly told to just *try* sex or somehow change our inclinations, because it shouldn't be a big deal to just test it out and see.

To see it from our perspective, let's say you're a heterosexual person. Say every time you say so, people ask you why you don't try being "open-minded" enough to just try sex with your own gender. They tell you you're missing out and refuse to take you seriously if you're not willing to experiment. Do most people feel this is an inappropriate request? Probably. Would most heterosexual people be able to be "reasoned into" trying sex with their own gender just in the interest of remaining open-minded? Probably not.

Please understand that it might feel like sex isn't really a big deal if it's not a big deal to *you*, but for someone who doesn't feel that attraction, "just trying it" might very well be too much to ask. (Especially since, in our experience, we just get told we did it wrong or with the wrong person if we try it and still don't like it.) "Just try it" sounds unreasonable to many of us—perhaps as unreasonable as "just go without it, it's no big deal" would sound to people who value and pursue sex. There are asexual people who have sex, and they do so for various reasons (discussed in Part Two of this book), but for much of the population, a desire for sex grows out of being attracted to someone. Not being sexually attracted to anyone tends to strongly affect interest in seeking out sex for many people.

If you can't imagine yourself having sex with someone you're not attracted to (based on anything from gender to age to body type), you probably feel the way many asexual

> "Telling people they have to engage in unwanted sex before you consider their desires valid is a form of social coercion. It creates pressure on them to engage in unwanted sex, and it contributes to rape culture."
> —AYDAN SELBY, *THE ASEXUAL AGENDA*

people do when it comes to willingness to try it anyway. Remember that they might feel about having *any* sex the way you may feel about having sex with people you aren't sexually attracted to, and asexual people are unlikely to see you as an ally if you tell them they "should" be indifferent enough to experiment. **Asexual people don't have an obligation to try to be otherwise, and that's really important to remember when talking about our orientation with us.** You'll be establishing a double standard if you don't expect most people to try multiple types and genders of partners before they're trusted to label themselves, but that we, on the other hand, should try every other possibility before self-identifying as asexual. You'll have trouble getting us to take you seriously as an ally if you think we can only be asexual if we've tried and failed to be everything else.

Don't assume an asexual person in a romantic relationship must have decided to identify as asexual because a partner is bad at sex. This is especially important if you *are* the partner here and a significant other has recently revealed they are asexual. Remember this is not their way of saying a partner disappointed them in bed, or that they must not love their partner, or that a poor lover "made them asexual" (which no one can do, any more than anyone can make them change to any other sexual orientation), or that there is anything at all a person can do or could have done to stop them from coming to the conclusion that they are asexual.

Don't start setting down conditions for "belief" if an asexual person comes out—such as agreeing to believe them if they try dating and don't like it, claiming their orientation will be "proved" if they still don't want sex a year from now, or saying you'll believe them if they're still saying this when they're twenty-five. When your asexual friend or family member reveals their orientation to you, it does not mean you are being asked to intervene. You're not being asked for advice and you're not being recruited; you're just being asked to understand. **This isn't about putting yourself in an asexual person's shoes; it's about recognizing that people wear different shoes because they have different feet.**

If the only context you have for not having sex is wanting it but not getting it, you might have trouble with the idea of not getting it because you don't want it. An asexual person's life is not likely to be empty if it lacks sex, so if this is the only way you can see it—if it seems bleak and boring and horrific to you—then you are not processing this person's situation. You're processing *yourself* in a situation that would be distasteful to you, and until you accept that this is someone else's "normal," you may be unable to react constructively.

Don't tell the asexual person that you think asexuality awareness shouldn't be a big deal. Sometimes we hear remarks about how it's silly to want more visibility or how it's absurd to want to be part of a Pride parade or queer-related event.[1] We're often told it's no big deal because "so you don't want to have sex, so what? Nobody cares." If you've read the rest of this book, you know "not wanting to have sex" is both oversimplifying and misrepresenting asexuality, and in our experience, "nobody cares" is untrue. We deal with misguided interventions, aggressive questioning, and mocking (just for starters!) on a level that suggests a great need for more education on this topic.

Don't tell the asexual person that their terminology or identity is "too complicated." As mentioned previously, people tend to think asexuality is a very

---

1 "And then you have the asexuals marching for the right to not . . . do anything. Which is hilarious. You didn't need to march for that right. You just need to stay home and not do anything." —Dan Savage in the documentary *(A)sexual.* (Tucker, 2011)

simple concept, but when it's discussed in any depth, it becomes clear how nuanced and layered it can be. Sometimes we're painted as unreasonable if we expect others to understand identities like "gray-polyromantic demisexual," but we should expect asexuality to be complicated, since mainstream sexuality only seems less complicated because we're all used to it and have been hearing and understanding the contexts for those relationships since we were children. It's all right if you don't understand, especially if the asexual person uses many unfamiliar terms, but it's better if you either try to learn their terms or just say nothing. It won't be well received if you claim the orientation is too complicated for any reasonable person to learn about.

Don't immediately express doubts that the person is asexual (especially in the form of "but you have a partner!" or "but you want/have children!"), and **don't** ask the person to prove the validity of asexuality to you. This is also not the time to suggest that it would be better to try harder to be something else.

Don't worry about it if you have a really hard time getting your head around how a person could be asexual or what their experience must be like. Chances are they can't imagine sexual attraction either. You don't need to express how absolutely bizarre it may sound to you—expressing that may alienate the asexual person—and it's best that you **don't** joke that you'd *die* without sex or point out how much you value sex and sexuality in your life. It's okay for you to not get it; plenty of people don't. Just be respectful about it, the same as you should be if a person doesn't like a food you like.

And while we do want your acknowledgment if we're revealing this aspect of our lives to you, **don't** constantly bring it up in group settings or one-on-one chats. This often makes us feel like you can't think of us as anything but "that *asexual* person." We want it to be acknowledged as important, but we want it to be considered just one part of who we are to you, like your sexual orientation isn't the first thing on our minds when we talk to you. You may want to ask us whether we're out to the public about our asexuality because accidentally outing your friend or family member could be a disaster for both of you.

Somebody Just Told Me They're Asexual! What Do I Say?

Unfortunately, reactions usually come out sounding negative, even if they aren't meant that way; we often hear condescending utterances of "are you sure?" and "don't you think you'll regret that?" along with immediate laughter and denial ("ha, no you're not!") or attitudes ranging from disbelieving to horrified.

If someone comes out to you and you can't think of anything to say at first, try one of these:

- Thank the asexual person for sharing and for trusting you. Ask whether they have anything more they'd like to tell you about it.
- Ask the asexual person to tell you about how they discovered their asexuality if that's something they're interested in sharing. Discuss romantic orientation and what terms and labels they use to identify themselves if that would be a comfortable subject.
- Say something that suggests support for the idea of asexuality, such as saying you've heard of it, acknowledging that there have surely been asexual people throughout history, or that you think it only makes sense that some people in the world would be asexual. Acknowledging that it's just one more kind of normal is comforting.

This is the time to let the asexual person control the conversation. The asexual person may have been gearing up for the de-closeting for months, and there may be quite a lot of nerves involved . . . it's possible the asexual person has been preparing, and if you have been chosen to hear this message, your reaction probably means a lot. Make it a good one.

But What If I've Already Said Something Kind of Regrettable?

Well, that's understandable, especially if the idea of asexuality was really mind-blowing to you and you were either just so floored by the thought of asexual people or you were immediately anxious about what it meant for your friend or family member. The fact that you are reading a book about it does suggest that you want to be on board as an informed person in the asexual person's life, so that's a good place to start.

If you accidentally subjected the asexual person to a reaction you now regret, if appropriate, bring up the subject with the asexual person and say you're sorry for saying whatever you said. This will generally go over well if you follow the apology by saying you researched asexuality and that you had no idea there was so much information on the subject or that so many people feel this way. Acknowledge what you said or did as a knee-jerk reaction or a typical response considering the lack of education on asexuality in our culture, though you should try to avoid making it sound like an excuse.

You may wish to acknowledge that you were never taught about asexuality and that you now see why awareness efforts are so important. As soon as you tell an asexual person that you think more people need to know about the reality of their orientation, you will establish yourself as a clear ally. It would mean the world if you apologized to an asexual person you may have hurt and said "I just wish this had been discussed in sex ed." Yes, it should have been. The more non-asexual allies backing us up, the more likely it is that one day we *will* see it in our sexual education classrooms and textbooks.

Also, if the asexual person in question was rude to you when you didn't understand, treated you like you were a terrible person, or mocked you even though you don't think you did anything wrong, it's possible you're hearing the anger and annoyance that comes from years of frustration and repression. Asexual people are not exempt from behaving poorly sometimes, and it's possible someone was unfair to you, got angry at you very quickly for what seemed like an innocent question, or expected too much of you. It happens.

But remember, some negative emotions are understandable in our situation, and if an asexual person reacts snidely to your interest or your questions, the best thing you can do is educate yourself on your own. Many asexual people get tired of educating others and may be hostile if you press the issue, and the worst thing you can do is claim that you can't expect to learn if they won't personally educate you. A strong reaction suggests strong feelings, so it would be inappropriate to scold them for "overreacting" or to blame your inability to understand on their failure to be as calm as you are. They have more at stake when their identity is challenged and mocked, and the prevailing attitude toward asexuality in the mainstream has a real effect on their lives, so emotion-free levelheadedness is not always an option.

If the person who has reacted strongly is someone whose feelings matter to you, you can help by learning about asexuality and then reassuring them that you understand better now and won't bring it up unless they do. (You might consider a letter to express this if the person stays angry with you.)

You might not understand why they're upset, and maybe they really are being a bit unreasonable, but if you can make it clear you're an ally, not an adversary, they may come around. Understanding the reason behind their reaction may help, too. For instance, if you asked about their personal medical history or brought up possible abuse in their past, and they flew off the handle in response and refused to address it, you may not understand why such a simple question provoked an outburst. However, if you read the parts of this book that address those misconceptions (Part Three), you may get a feel for the context they may see these questions in.

They may perceive intent to harm or dismiss them if you choose certain phrases in your quest to understand more. Arguing about your true intent isn't wise if the asexual person was hurt by your words or actions regardless. You should also refrain from suggesting they or their cause will never gain ground if they're not nice enough. Do your best to figure out what triggered the negative reaction, and undo the damage if you can through apology, correcting yourself, or acknowledging that you don't understand. There may be times when you won't know why they responded to you the way they did, but try reading more about asexual people's experiences. If you begin to see what our world is like, you may at least find an explanation for said behavior, even if you don't think that explanation excuses it.

What If My Child Just Said They're Asexual? Are They Too Young to Know?

If you're the parent of an asexual teenager or adult, first off, it's great that you're seeking out a book on your child's experience. With the help of your child and other resources like this book, I hope you come to a good understanding of the orientation.

The mean age of the first sexual attraction experience is ten years old.[2] By the teenage years, children are typically very familiar with the concept of viewing other people sexually and finding them attractive. It's very unusual to reach late teenagerhood without feeling sexual attraction or sexual inclination at all, and if that is what your child is reporting, it's possible they are asexual.

Of course, yes, there are other possibilities that could be at work: health issues, social anxiety, embarrassment, fear of consequences like sexually transmitted infections and pregnancy, latent or hidden homosexuality, fear of dating, off-putting experiences, lack of available partners, et cetera. But what exactly is your child saying? Are they invoking a circumstantial reason for not wanting to date or have sex, or are they saying "I don't find anyone sexually attractive"? If it is the latter, that's what asexuality is. If they're labeling themselves "asexual" at this point but you believe one of these other possibilities is more likely, it's still best not to say so, because they may feel invalidated and less willing to share their problems and feelings in the future.

Asexuality is very unlikely to indicate a health issue in and of itself. Health problems that cause disinterest in sex have other symptoms (discussed fully in a subsection of Part Three), and if you are still making your child's health decisions, you shouldn't take your child to a medical or mental health professional deliberately trying to "cure" them of asexuality. As a responsible parent, you will of course

---

2 "Recent findings from three distinct and significant studies have pointed to the age of 10 as the mean age of first sexual attraction—well before puberty." (McClintock & Herdt, 1996)

be concerned about the health of your child, but perhaps it's best to research sexual-desire-related disorders and try to understand what you can expect to see if your child does have a problem. If you do converse with your child about personal problems or take them to a counselor, try to avoid implying that you're arranging an intervention to fix asexuality as a problem. Even if they are not asexual but are trying out the label, they will cooperate more willingly with you and with professionals if their exploration is respected, not immediately dismissed as impossible.

That said, telling your child "you'll grow out of it" or "you're not old enough to decide that yet" may very deeply hurt or frustrate them. You may even be **right** that they are going through a phase—some people do experiment with identity when trying to figure out their attractions and what labels to use—but it will not be helpful in the slightest if you announce you do not accept what they're feeling as valid and believe yourself to be the authority on what they could possibly be experiencing.

Many asexual people know they're asexual when they're in their young teens—because when everyone else is figuring out who they are attracted to, asexual teens are realizing they aren't attracted to anyone. Even if they are

> "Having someone tell you 'Hey it's ok to feel that way!' makes such a big difference. (. . .) If someone grows a bit and realizes that they do experience sexual attraction or does like sex, that's ok! And they may, more likely than not, have an easier time coming to that conclusion and accepting it than if they reached that conclusion from a place of shame and ridicule."
> —Fiish

indeed wrong about being asexual, announcing that you *do not believe them* may alienate your child and cause them to be less likely to include you in their personal thoughts and identity exploration in the future. There are ways to be supportive and reserve judgment even if you privately think your child may choose a different label later in life, and it's likely they'll be more willing to trust you in their relationship issues as they grow if you establish yourself as a parent willing to listen. If it's true that they will "grow out of it" or change their label later, they will do so regardless of whether you've told them they will.

What If My Partner Just Said They're Asexual? What Do I Do?

This happens fairly often. People who are already in marriages or other long-term relationships suddenly (or so it seems) start identifying as asexual and want to change the game. What should you do, as a non-asexual person who's found themselves in a relationship with an asexual person?

It's not unusual for a partnership that includes a mixture of non-asexual and asexual people to undergo some stress. If you are a non-asexual partner, you may wonder why this had to come up when everything seemed okay before—if in fact it did seem okay. You may feel cheated or hurt or worried that an asexual partner is now going to remove sex from the relationship—or that they never fully loved you, or that they were lying if they had sex with you despite their lack of attraction. It's normal to feel hurt if they did not share an important aspect of their feelings toward you.

But remember: asexual people who have never heard of their own orientation are trained since childhood to think sex is an unavoidable part of all romantic relationships and that no one will love them without it (or, in some cases, they think their love must be fractured somehow if it does not make them feel sexual attraction). **Asexual people are taught to hide it if they don't feel what everybody else seems to feel.** The way things were before may not have been okay with them, but they were conditioned not to speak of such an alien experience as *not being sexually attracted* to the partner they love so much.

They may have felt too ashamed or confused to share these feelings, may have been worried you'll think they want to break up, or that you'll think it's your fault for not being sexy to them. Until they discovered the existence of asexuality, they very well may have thought they were the only person to feel this way, and that's hard to say out loud.

> "Sexual scripts are not second nature. We are aware of them (have seen the same movies and read the same books as you have) but the common tropes in these stories do not represent our experience. We may have assumed that these tropes are purely fiction, that nobody actually feels that way, that everyone feels the way we do, rather than suspect that we are the odd ones out. Many of us are familiar enough with sexual scripts to use them in conversation, but we treat them like jokes or figures of speech."
> —REBECCA, *SEIJI HAS MANY SOCKS*

So if an asexual partner comes out to you and wants to renegotiate certain aspects of your sex life or your relationship, don't blame yourself for supposed bad sex, don't take it as a sign that you are not an attractive person, and don't beat yourself up over it if the prospect of having to change your sex life to accommodate an asexual partner's needs is intimidating to you. Sometimes partners determine that their needs are indeed too different to stay together, and there's no shame in that; however, there are many different compromises that can be reached, and some of them can be better understood by reading Part Two of this book under "Asexual Relationships."

In any case, you're now going forward. You have to figure out how to negotiate this relationship. While doing so, keep in mind that this is going to involve compromise if you're going to stay together, and furthermore, compromise is not something only meant for the asexual partner(s). Try to see your relationship as having "mismatched sexual desires or needs" rather than "they don't want sex enough." You may have incompatible desires, but a compromise is possible in many cases. You may be able to examine your boundaries and desires and figure out whether you can compromise by making a list of must-haves and dealbreakers, either on your own or by using a resource to guide you.[3]

Some asexual people enjoy sex. Some are indifferent or ambivalent toward it. Some are repulsed. If your asexual partner(s) said sex is completely off the table as a bargaining item, you should listen and understand they are serious. And if, when you deeply examine your feelings, you realize that you cannot be romantic, intimate, or committed with anyone who does not want to have sex (or feels differently about it than you thought they did), it's okay to recognize that you need your partner to desire you the way you desire them.

No one should ever feel *obligated* to have sex, so please do not ever treat someone like they are betraying an automatic requirement or expectation in all relationships. But no one should have to remain in a relationship that isn't what they thought it was and includes a dealbreaker, either. If you're honest and say you won't be able to live with that, you're not any more in the wrong than an asexual partner who says they can't live with being expected to have or to want sex. You are free to leave the relationship if it is best for both of you . . . and if you are indeed so mismatched that you absolutely require something an asexual partner is absolutely unwilling to give, it's probably best.

However, if your asexual partner(s) would be willing to start or continue to have occasional or regular sex, you will still have to negotiate how often, what kind of sex, and under what circumstances. Make sure you're honest about your feelings, including your dealbreakers, your must-haves, and whatever aspects of your relationship are up for compromise, and be sure to check and double-check for understanding both when you're first forming your terms and when you've been living with them for a while.

---

3 Checklists can be used or modified from the resources at *Scarleteen* (www.scarleteen.com/article/ advice/yes_no_maybe_so_a_sexual_inventory_stocklist) or *SmartHotFun* (smarthotfun.com/ wantwillwontchart).

Some asexual people may be willing to engage in only certain kinds of sex, focus on sensual instead of sexual experiences, or involve toys, kinks, fetishes, or other practices. Some asexual people don't mind or enjoy manual stimulation with their partners or watching their partners stimulate themselves. And relationship-wise, some asexual people are willing to change the terms of a previously two-person partnership to include open relationships[4] or polyamory,[5] so partners can satisfy unmet needs without its being "cheating."

If you're dedicated to staying with a partner who is asexual, it's possible you actually don't think lack of sex would be a big deal for you. Maybe you're willing to go without sex, or take care of any sexual arousal yourself, and if that's the case, you should discuss it with your asexual partner(s). But also feel free to be honest if you try it for a while and it's just not working. After all, if you come to a sexual compromise and they eventually determine that they need to revise "what's allowed," they should be able to tell you; you should feel the same amount of freedom to let a significant other know what you're feeling and what you need and figure out how to meet your needs together.

But even if you're breaking up over a partner's asexuality, you should never suggest an asexual partner will never find someone who will accept them except another asexual person. Relationships between asexual people and non-asexual people do work sometimes on all sorts of compatibility issues, and the key is always communication and compromise. Never imply to an asexual person that lack of willingness to have sex makes them "damaged goods," or that relationships are "about" sex, or that it's not real love unless it involves sex, period. Asexual people do hear suggestions like these in relationships sometimes, and these messages strip asexual people of their confidence and self-worth. You do need to remember to only speak for yourself about what you want in a partner. Other people do exist who can have happy relationships with asexual people, and you shouldn't try to convince others that they do not exist.

Here are some suggestions for how to have a happy relationship with an asexual person, beyond just discussing your basic dealbreakers and must-haves:

- Communicate about your signals for intimacy. Do you have certain hints, signs, or terms for how you tell each other what you want? Try to remember that some non-asexual people you may have previously dated might

---

4 Open relationships are non-monogamous relationships wherein a couple stays committed to each other but one or both parties will be allowed to take other partners.

5 Polyamory refers to a type of open relationship wherein one or more of the partners have an intimate relationship with more than one person, generally with mutually agreed-upon terms. This could involve one or more partners having another partner *or* can include triad or group-partner situations.

have used certain behaviors to initiate sex, while your asexual partner(s) may not mean the same thing. "What does it mean when you say/do X? How would you rather I respond?" is a good way to start this conversation.

- Focus on the aspects of your relationship that make it so special—the aspects that make it different from your friendships or other important relationships. Why are you partners? What can you do together that you don't do with anyone else? Heighten and celebrate these if it helps you remain close to your partner(s).

- Don't assume the asexual partner(s) would prefer to stop all physical or sensual activities just because sex might be absent or non-traditional. Communicate about what types of touch you would like to enjoy together; plenty of sensual activities are possible and worthwhile even if they don't lead to sex.

- Understand that your asexual partner(s) may not connect sex and romance in their own desires. If you normally would have sex to celebrate an anniversary, to express thanks for something they did for you, or to enhance the enjoyment of an intimate date, try to communicate about whether that is appropriate with the asexual partner(s) and under what circumstances sex *is* connected to other aspects of your romance (if any).

- Be willing to acknowledge asexuality in conversations about your relationship with third parties. If your asexual partner(s) can be comfortable with being "out" to others, treating this relationship like it's just one more normal way to be intimate with a certain kind of person may be welcomed. Being an open ally is a great way to show support, and it fosters trust.

- If sex is still something you and your asexual partner(s) plan to do, ask if they'd be more comfortable with clearly defined days, times, and situations in which sex will take place. Many non-asexual people rely on picking up innuendo or sexual cues, whereas some asexual people might not feel that these cues actually are a signal for sex. Depending on their ability to read you and your previously built trust, you may need to be verbal about it, and it's better to say "I'm in the mood, how do you feel about going to the bedroom?" than to just initiate a backrub or something similar and hope it leads to sex, ultimately possibly being disappointed if it doesn't. If you don't want to schedule sexual activities, you may suggest your asexual partner(s) wear or say or do something if they want to initiate or would be willing to accept sex.

- Don't assume that if an asexual partner enjoys sex, they must want you to do more or do it more often than you'd agreed upon. What might seem an enthusiastic response and a request for "more" from most people might not be that at all from an asexual partner. Always ask your partner what kinds of responses they'd appreciate.

- Try not to be offended if you suggest sex and they don't want to. Sometimes it's easier for an asexual person to process and get "warmed up" for having sex if they have time to think about it for an hour or a day, so if your partner(s) would be open to this, discuss whether it'd be appropriate to leave a note or a text proposing what you'd like to do tonight. Some asexual people respond better to that than they do to what seems to them a sudden come-on. If they say no even in this situation, you may ask whether asking that way was okay and see if they still want you to try again another time. Never behaving as if it's just expected will usually result in more "yes" answers.

- If you seek counseling, don't approach it as if the asexuality is something your partner(s) can or should "get over," and don't just pretend to be understanding about their situation while secretly assuming they'll go back to how it was before once they work through issues.

- Take care to communicate with the asexual partner(s) and reassure them that they aren't a disappointment. Most asexual people will worry for a long time that you're secretly hoping for more from them or that you will get fed up over your mismatched sexual needs. If this is not the case, telling them how you feel will help more than you know.

- If a certain kind of touch makes your asexual partner(s) uncomfortable or falls solidly into the "sexual" category for them *even if you don't think it does*, discuss when and whether these touches and actions would be welcomed or allowed. Never try to convince them that something you want to do (e.g., innocently grabbing their butt or going naked at home) is not in fact sexual and therefore they "should" be open to it, and especially never tell them what they should be willing to do if they want to prove they love you.

- Your partner(s) may have nonsexual needs that you can satisfy, and you should try to understand that these may be just as important, persistent, real, and intense as your sexual needs are. (In other words, sexual needs do not outrank all other needs in a relationship, and their needs shouldn't be regarded as something to be ignored until or unless yours are satisfied.) All partners should be able to discuss their greatest needs and how they want them satisfied, and they should be approached with the attitude of wanting to have a loving relationship, not in a bargain-based atmosphere of humoring one another or grudgingly giving in order to receive.

Also, keep in mind that people may criticize your relationship if your partner(s) will be coming out to others in your family or social circle. In dealing with the criticism, you may feel mocked for being in a relationship with an asexual person, especially if others believe you are shamefully "not getting any" or being submissive by "caving" to an asexual person's possibly lower sexual allowances. Especially if you are a man, your fitness as a person or a partner may be attacked or questioned.

People may try to encourage you to leave the asexual partner(s) or tell you that you could do better, or they may just be very curious about how your relationship works and ask you intrusive questions about your sex life or each of your genitals. They may

> "The host (. . .) says to my boyfriend, 'So, I heard you were asexual. What's that about?' My boyfriend had to explain that I was asexual, but he wasn't. This led to a situation where all his friends were quizzing him on asexuality. My boyfriend felt very uncomfortable because he felt put on the spot to defend the legitimacy of our relationship to his friends."
> —TRISTAN MILLER, *THE ASEXUAL AGENDA*

heap unsolicited advice upon you about what you should "try" to change the asexual person. Note that this more often happens when your asexual partner(s) cannot be there to witness it. You can combat this by checking with your asexual partner(s) about what's okay to say about your relationship, and if you'd rather not do asexual-relationship-Q&A, choose one or two affirming sentences to address criticism. Express happiness with your relationship or tell detractors that it's not their business, and repeat it until they stop asking.

If you do choose to stay with your partner(s), you may find some comfort in a) checking out resources for non-asexual partners of asexual people in forums such as the *Asexual Visibility and Education Network* (www.asexuality.org); b) reading through the misconceptions section of this book (Part Three) to find rebuttals and deconstructions for the questions and comments people make; and c) reading through the "if you're asexual" section of this book (Part Four) to learn what asexual people face and how to be a better supporter and ally for them.

Can I Ask Questions?

This, again, varies greatly by individual. If an asexual person has done something awareness-related in a public forum and you are interacting with that asexual person through the public forum, questions are usually appropriate and even welcomed. Many asexual awareness activists are quite used to being asked out-and-out crude questions, so your polite ones are unlikely to offend us. Use a little more caution when you're talking to someone who's discussing the subject with you one on one.

And you can't go wrong if you politely *ask* if you can ask first. Some people will just say "Sorry, I don't really want to talk about my personal life." You can still find the answers to general questions by interacting through forums (some discussion groups are listed in the References section of this book) or submitting your request to an asexuality-related Q&A blog.[6]

Some asexual people just want to be asexual people, not spokespeople. As with any underrepresented population, we are often portrayed as being representative of "our group," so please keep in mind that we don't necessarily speak for each other and that our answers are not to be generalized as the accepted status quo for "the community."

What Questions Can I Ask Without Making Someone Uncomfortable?

We would like your questions to be open-minded, polite, and not rendered in biased language. For instance, a question like "Don't you think you'd better get your hormone levels checked?" is stacked toward "of course you should." If you really want to know whether the asexual person in question might have a hormonal issue, keep in mind that's a personal medical question and it may very well not be your business. Also keep in mind that hormonal lack of sex drive is different from lack of sexual attraction, and if someone has a disorder, there are observable health problems that develop from it. (There is more about that in Part Three of this book, which discusses asexuality's being mistaken for a disorder.) We frequently hear these kinds of questions about health from well-meaning people as well as from people who are trying to knock us down on purpose.

So imagine you're talking to a person who is the same sexual orientation you are. Then ask yourself whether you are close enough to that person to say such things as "Say, do your genitals work?" or "Do you masturbate?" or "Have you ever had an orgasm?" In some people's minds, these kinds of questions suddenly become fair game to ask asexual strangers or acquaintances when people want to know how we function.

---

6 Try *Asexual Advice*, a blog that takes submissions either through Tumblr accounts or anonymously: asexualadvice.tumblr.com.

Asking these questions is not recommended unless your relationship with that person is such that you could have comfortably asked the same questions if the person wasn't asexual. (Meaning *they* would be comfortable too!) We generally don't like being thrown impersonally under the microscope and used for answer mining. If you suddenly switch into "but the specimen exists to satisfy my curiosity!" mode, don't be surprised if that person withdraws from you as a result. If you treat people impersonally and behave as if they owe you answers, they will withdraw.

Anything I Should Avoid Assuming?

Yes. Here are some worries that might be bothering you about asexual people and your relationship with an asexual friend or loved one.

Asexual people aren't looking down on you for your sexuality. Some people automatically believe

> "I feel as if any movement that claims to be about sexual freedom as a whole that almost solely concerns itself with the issues of people with average-to-high sexual desire is going to be missing vital issues, and that it will often end in new sexual obligations and norms. I think sex-positivity needs asexuality, needs to talk about this side of the coin and the issues people face here."
>
> —Kaz, *Feministe*

that if someone's asexual, it constitutes taking a stand against sex (necessitating defense of or adamant glorification of one's sexuality), and that is not the case at all.

Many asexual people who don't want to have sex still support consensual sexual relationships, as long as the sex doesn't involve them. Empowerment regarding sex should always include the option to *not* engage in it. Unfortunately, some folks in sex-positive movements misinterpret sex positivity as "sex is good, period," and this can be turned against asexual people. If a sex-positive person thinks the only way to celebrate sex is to encourage more of it, that person may believe asexual people who choose to abstain are doing so because of a sex-negative attitude. Sex positivity isn't about shaming people for not having enough sex. If you want to put forward a sex-positive message, keep this in mind when you choose your words. Make it about freedom, not about demonizing those who don't feel interested or accusing them of internalized oppression. If someone is sex positive, their message should be about choice—about not marginalizing anyone based on lifestyle or inclination, even if said lifestyle includes no sex at all.

Abstinent asexual people might sometimes be relieved that they don't have some of the problems sex causes, but they have a whole different set of problems, and they don't think of themselves as superior. They just want to be respected. Asexual people are generally okay with sex being a big part of other people's lives, and they're not trying to take it away from anyone. Asexual people also don't need to hear about how much a sexually active person enjoys their sex life, as if this will make asexual people feel insecure about what they might be missing and "reconsider." Asexual people are not judging anyone for wanting sex or enjoying it or celebrating it.

Remember we aren't necessarily disgusted by or naive about relationships or sexuality. *Asexual* is not a synonym for *sex negative* or *dateless*. Sometimes people bend over backwards to placate their one asexual guest, trying to avoid references to sex in conversation, or deliberately leaving their asexual friend out of an invitation to a movie that features romance or sexual situations. Unless we've expressed that we wish to be left out, please don't assume "oh that would gross you out," and also don't assume that we have no idea how sex or dating works. Many of us date/have dated and some of us have had sex/ are sexually active, and nearly all of us are going to know the facts of life. Don't censor yourself or feel that you have to explain to the wide-eyed innocent. It's unlikely that we're at all mystified by the workings of sexual relationships if we have typical understandings of other social relationships.

We aren't buying into a fad or trying to be unique. This may sound silly, but ask any asexual person who's done visibility work and they'll tell you they've heard these multiple times: "You just want attention" or "Everybody's trying to be special these days" or "This is silly; why do you need a label for all the sex you're *not* having?"

> "The asexual community generally tries to facilitate people figuring themselves out. Introspection, and detailed analysis is fashionable. There's active discussion about what it means to be between asexual and non-asexual. People feel free to express their doubts. There's a lot of uncertainty involved in asexuality, but asexuals deal with it in healthy ways. What's unhealthy is the way that everyone else constantly questions the validity of asexuality upon first encountering it. Somehow it fails to fit in their worldview, and people just deny deny deny."
>
> —TRISTAN MILLER, SKEPTIC'S PLAY

Asexuality isn't "a fad" any more than homosexuality was a fad when the number of "out" gay people increased significantly. The LGBTQ movement's awareness efforts led, in part, to the formation of safe spaces for LGBTQ people, and the more visible they became, the more people felt comfortable coming out. Asexual people are much rarer than gay people, and since society constantly hits us over the head with "of course we're all compelled by sex" messages, we know our feelings are unpopular. If there weren't Internet-based communities, most of us would probably be the only asexual person we'd ever heard of. And while awareness of a phenomenon does trigger some misapplied labeling, it'd be extremely offensive to write off everyone who comes out as asexual. It's unlikely that we'd read about it on the Internet and think "that's me!" if we'd never had an inkling of the sort before.

Asexuality isn't a decision, an oath, or a phase. For most of us, saying we're asexual is just like anyone else declaring their sexual orientation. But we acknowledge that things do sometimes change and we are sometimes wrong about ourselves, just like people of any sexual orientation are. It isn't fair to treat asexual people as though our orientation is temporary, but keep in mind being asexual is not the same as having sworn off sex.

If we are telling you we're asexual, we're stating a fact about how we feel; asexuality is not a logical decision based on close-mindedness that you have to reason with us about. In short, you aren't going to change our attraction experiences by arguing that we won't have a full life unless we "change our minds." We haven't made a decision. We've made an observation, and we're living our lives based on the assumption that what we've observed about ourselves is true.

Some of us do have sex and/or experience nonsexual attractions to other people, and you should never point to these facts as "evidence" that we cannot actually be asexual. There are reasons to have sex besides sexual attraction, and some people are sexually intimate for those reasons. There are other ways to be attracted to others—romantically, sensually, aesthetically— and they aren't half-formed or stunted sexual attractions "trying" to come out, so it shouldn't be assumed that they invalidate our identity. The romantic relationships and non-romantic relationships that asexual people have should be described and respected using the terms they themselves use, and their ability to determine what kind of relationship they have should be trusted. Types of asexual partnerships and the terms we use are discussed extensively in Part Two.

And as a final thought: **please remember that a big part of being an ally is being one even when no asexual people are there to appreciate it.**

We don't want to recruit you for an advertising campaign, but if you're allied with our visibility efforts, you can help in a natural way. Do what you can as far as research on the subject so you don't end up spreading misinformation, and if you see or hear a conversation that misrepresents, erases, or mocks asexual people/asexuality, say something. If you study sexuality or are in some way devoted to increasing awareness about its many facets, make sure you include asexuality in a realistic capacity—as in, don't give it its own special section and then go back to discussing sexuality as if there's no such thing. We're not asking you to play advocate if that's not something you'd do regarding any other type of misinformation, but if that IS something you enjoy, we're happy to have you helping us spread awareness.

PART SIX:
OTHER RESOURCES

H ere are some supplementary resources that can help you research asexuality, talk to asexual people, read personal accounts, understand the subject, or network with others. Please note that the resources mentioned here are primarily accessible on the Internet and may contain contradictory or controversial opinions.

Basic Information, Introductions, Organizations, and FAQs:

- **The Asexual Visibility and Education Network (AVEN):**
  "*AVEN* hosts the world's largest online asexual community as well as a large archive of resources on asexuality."
  http://asexuality.org

- **Asexual Awareness Week:**
  "Asexual Awareness Week is an international organization dedicated to raising awareness and visibility about the asexual spectrum worldwide."
  http://asexualawarenessweek.com/

- **Partnership for Asexual Visibility and Education (PAVE):**
  "Our goal is different than other asexuality projects. This project aims to mobilize aces and allies across the United States with shared political values to take action for progressive policy issues, including asexual issues."
  http://acesandallies.org/

- **Asexual Resources and Education (ARE:UK):**
  "The organisation provides resources for asexuals, allies and others such as teachers and healthcare workers whilst working with academics to increase understanding and acceptance of asexuality in professional sectors."
  http://www.are-uk.com/

- **Asexuality–The Student Room:**
  "Have you ever wondered what it means when someone says they are asexual? This article lays out some of the common questions that you might have about asexuality and then answers them for you."
  http://www.thestudentroom.co.uk/wiki/Asexuality

- **AVEN Project Team:**
  "A group of members dedicated to overseeing *AVEN's* many efforts to bring education and visibility to the outside world."
  http://avenpt.tumblr.com/

- **Asexuality Archive:**
  "*The Asexuality Archive* is a collection of all things Ace. In these pages, I hope to provide a comprehensive and uncensored look into what asexuality is, what it means to us and how it shapes our lives. My intention is to provide information that is approachable and informative, whether or not you're asexual."
  Site: http://www.asexualityarchive.com/
  Book: http://www.asexualityarchive.com/book/

- **The Asexual Agenda:**
  "*The Asexual Agenda* has two primary goals: 1. Stimulate and promote asexual blogs. We serve as a community center: a place for readers to discuss with each other, and a portal to other asexual blogs. 2. Strive towards greater understanding, especially in our target audience: people under the ace spectrum who already understand the basics."
  http://asexualagenda.wordpress.com

- **Asexuality Resources:**
  A collection of helpful links to other places on the web, including YouTube videos, Tumblr essays, asexual people's blogs, and research.
  http://juliesondradecker.com/?page_id=2058

- **Asexual Advice:**
  This blog takes submissions from readers, using a team of volunteer asexual people who are experienced in answering questions.
  http://asexualadvice.tumblr.com/

Discussion Groups, Networking, and Forums

- **The Asexual Visibility and Education Network Forums:**
  AVEN's forums to discuss all aspects of asexuality—open to asexual people and allies.
  http://www.asexuality.org/en/

- **The Tumblr Asexual Community:**
  Hundreds of bloggers use the #asexual tag to discuss issues. (Unmoderated, so can contain misinformation and trolls, but lots of networking and connection is possible on Tumblr.)
  http://www.tumblr.com/tagged/asexual

- **The Asexuality LiveJournal Group:**
  "This is a community for asexual people to discuss living without sexuality. We welcome anyone with no or very little sexual attraction to others, people with low or no libido, and their allies."
  http://asexuality.livejournal.com/

- **Asexual Groups:**
  "A catalog of all of the existing asexual communities around the world."
  http://asexualgroups.com/

- **Apositive:**
  "Apositive was developed to break new ground in discourse related to asexuality and sexuality."
  http://apositive.org/

- **Transyada:**
  An asexuality-friendly discussion forum with a focus on providing a space for people who identify as a non-binary gender or some form of transgender.
  http://transyada.net/forum/

- **Fetlife:**
  This fetish community is asexual-friendly and has support groups specifically for asexual people if they are kinksters.
  http://fetlife.com/groups/7247 (Asexual & Kinky)
  http://fetlife.com/groups/41247 (Ace BDSM Support Group)

- **AceFet:**
  This fetish community is specifically for asexual people with kinks.
  http://www.acefet.org/

- **Resources for Ace Survivors:**
  Asexual people who have experienced abuse or sexual assault can find support and help here.
  http://resourcesforacesurvivors.tumblr.com

- **The Asexuality Facebook Group:**
  Asexuality discussions of all kinds happen here.
  http://www.facebook.com/home.php?sk=group_2235733740

- **The AVEN Facebook Group:**
  AVEN's official group on Facebook.
  http://www.facebook.com/group.php?gid=2229697669

- **Acebook:**
  "*Acebook* is a unique dating and social networking site for asexual people."
  http://www.ace-book.net/index.php

Academic Resources and Research Collectives

- **Asexual Explorations:**
  "*Asexual Explorations* exists to promote the academic study of asexuality."
  http://www.asexualexplorations.net/home/

- **Asexuality Studies:**
  "Asexuality Studies is an online forum for asexuality research which was launched in October 2011."
  http://asexualitystudies.org/

- **The Asexual Sexologist:**
  "I created this page because I needed a place to start sorting through all of the resources I was finding while doing my research for my Masters in Human Sexuality (with a focus on Asexuality)."
  http://asexualsexologist.wordpress.com/

- **Understanding Asexuality:**
  "The time is right for a better understanding of this sexual orientation, written by an expert in the field who has conducted studies on asexuality and who has provided important contributions to understanding asexuality."
  Book by Anthony F. Bogaert, March 2012, ISBN 1442200995.

- **Asexualities: Feminist and Queer Perspectives (Routledge Research in Gender and Society):**
  "As the first book-length collection of critical essays ever produced on the topic of asexuality, this book serves as a foundational text in a growing field of study."
  Book by Megan Milks and Karli June Cerankowski, March 2014, ISBN 0415714427.

- **Asexuality and Sexual Normativity: An Anthology:**
  "This unique volume collects a diverse range of interdisciplinary empirical and theoretical work which addresses this emergence, raising important and timely questions about asexuality and its broader implications for sexual culture."
  Book by Mark Carrigan, Kristina Gupta, and Todd G. Morrison, May 2014, ISBN 0415731321.

Brochures and Educational Materials

- AVEN's materials:
  http://www.asexuality.org/en/topic/30115-official-aven-documents/

- Asexual Awareness Week's materials:
  http://www.asexualawarenessweek.com/resources.html

- Transcending Boundaries' materials:
  http://www.transcendingboundaries.org/pdf/asexuality_brochure.pdf

- Asex 101 with David Jay (slides and audio lecture):
  http://asexuality.org/wiki/index.php?title=Asex_101

Published Papers and Book Chapters on Asexuality

- "Asexuality as a Spectrum: A National Probability Sample Comparison to the Sexual Community in the UK." Caroline H. McClave, Master's Thesis, Columbia University, May 2013.
  http://academiccommons.columbia.edu/catalog/ac:162382
- "Intergroup Bias Toward 'Group X': Evidence of prejudice, dehumanization, avoidance, and discrimination against asexuals." Cara C. MacInnis & Gordon Hodson, *Group Processes & Intergroup Relations*, September 2012.
  http://gpi.sagepub.com/content/15/6/725
- "Producing facts: Empirical asexuality and the scientific study of sex." Ela Przybylo, *Feminism & Psychology*, 2012.
  http://fap.sagepub.com/content/early/2012/04/20/0959353512443668.abstract?rss=1
- "How Do You Know You Don't Like It If You Haven't Tried It?" Mark Carrigan, Chapter in *Sexual Minority Research in the New Millennium*, Todd G. Morrison, Melanie A. Morrison, Mark A. Carrigan, & Daragh T. McDermott, 2012, ISBN 1612099394.
- "Asexuality: An Emergent Sexual Orientation." Stephanie B. Gazzola & Melanie A. Morrison, Chapter in *Sexual Minority Research in the New Millennium*, Todd G. Morrison, Melanie A. Morrison, Mark A. Carrigan, & Daragh T. McDermott, 2012, ISBN 1612099394.
- "The Presence of Absence: Asexuality and the Creation of Resistance." Lily Hughes, *Gnovis Journal*, November 2011.
  http://gnovisjournal.org/2011/11/21/lily-hughes-journal
- "Furthering Our Understanding of Asexuality: An Investigation into Biological Markers of Asexuality, and the Development of the Asexuality Identification Scale." Morag Allison Yule, The University of British Columbia, August 2011.
  https://circle.ubc.ca/bitstream/id/131897/ubc_2011_fall_yule_morag.pdf
- "Physiological and Subjective Sexual Arousal in Self-Identified Asexual Women." Lori Brotto & Morag Allison Yule, *Archives of Sexual Behavior*, August 2011.
  http://www.obgyn.ubc.ca/SexualHealth/documents/Brotto%20&%20Yule%202011%20-Physiological%20&%20subjective%20sexual%20arousal%20in%20asexual%20women%20%7B%7B2675%7D%7D.pdf

- "Asexuality in disability narratives." Eunjung Kim, *Sexualities*, August 2011.
  http://sexualities.sagepub.com/content/14/4/479.abstract
- "Performing Asexuality through Narratives of Sexual Identity." Janet L. Sundrud, Master's Thesis, San José University, August 2011.
  http://scholarworks.sjsu.edu/cgi/viewcontent.cgi?article=5119&context=etd_theses
- "Asexual Scripts: A Grounded Theory Inquiry Into the Intrapsychic Scripts Asexuals Use to Negotiate Romantic Relationships." Carol Haefner, dissertation for a Doctorate of Philosophy at the Institute of Transpersonal Psychology, April 2011.
  http://gradworks.umi.com/3457969.pdf
- "There's more to life than sex? Difference and commonality within the asexual community." Mark A. Carrigan, *Sexualities*, 2011.
  http://sexualities.sagepub.com/content/14/4/462.abstract
- "Theoretical issues in the study of asexuality." CJ DeLuzio Chasin, *Archives of Sexual Behavior*, 2011.
  http://www.springerlink.com/content/g6qq605677372428/
- "Radical refusals: On the anarchist politics of women choosing asexuality." Breanne Fahs, *Sexualities*, August 2010.
  http://sex.sagepub.com/content/13/4/445.abstract
- "Asexuality: a mixed-methods approach." Lori Brotto, Gail Knudson, Jess Inskip; Katherine Rhodes; Yvonne Erskine, *Archives of Sexual Behavior*, June 2010.
  http://prod.obgyn.ubc.ca/SexualHealth/documents/Brotto%20et%20al.%202010-%20Asexuality%20...%20%7B%7B2206%7D%7D.pdf
- "What Asexuality Contributes to the Same-Sex Marriage Discussion." Kristin Scherrer, *Journal of Gay Lesbian Social Services*, January 2010.
  http://www.ncbi.nlm.nih.gov/pmc/articles/PMC2892980/
- "New Orientations: Asexuality and Its Implications for Theory and Practice." Karli Cerankowski & Megan Milks, *Feminist Studies*, 2010.
- "How much sex is healthy? The pleasures of asexuality." Eunjung Kim, Chapter in *Against Health: How Health Became the New Morality*, Jonathan M. Metzl & Anna Rutherford Kirkland, 2010, ISBN 0814795935.
- "Crisis and safety: The asexual in sexusociety." Ela Przybylo, *Sexualities*, 2010.
  http://sexualities.sagepub.com/content/14/4/444.abstract

- "Patterns of Asexuality in the United States." Dudley L. Poston, Jr. & Amanda K. Baumle, *Demographic Research*, 2010.
  http://www.demographic-research.org/volumes/vol23/18/23-18.pdf
- "Asexual Relationships: What Does Asexuality Have to Do with Polyamory?" Kristin S. Scherrer, Chapter in *Understanding Non-Monogamies* by Meg Barker & Darren Langdridge, 2009, ISBN 0415652960.
- "Coming to an Asexual Identity: Negotiating identity, negotiating desire." Kristin S. Scherrer, *Sexualities*, 2008.
  http://www.ncbi.nlm.nih.gov/pmc/articles/PMC2893352/
- "Asexuality: Dysfunction or variation." Anthony Bogaert, Chapter in *Psychological Sexual Dysfunctions* by Jayson M. Caroll & Marta K. Alena, 2008, ISBN 1604560487.
- "Asexuality: Classification and Clarification." Nicole Prause & Cynthia A. Graham, *Archives of Sexual Behavior*, 2007.
  http://www.kinseyinstitute.org/publications/PDF/PrauseGraham.pdf
- "Toward a Conceptual Understanding of Asexuality." Anthony Bogaert, *Review of General Psychology*, 2006.
- "Asexuality: Prevalence and Associated Factors in a National Probability Sample." Anthony Bogaert, *Journal of Sex Research*, 2004.
- "Asexual and Autoerotic Women: Two invisible groups." Myra T. Johnson, Chapter in *The Sexually Oppressed* by Jean S. Gochros and Harvey L. Gochros, 1977, ISBN 0809619156.

Published Articles and Interviews on Asexuality

Asexuality has been a topic of much discussion in the media—more and more frequently as it becomes more widely acknowledged. Various facets of the orientation have been explored in mainstream media throughout the years; articles and interviews have been featured in such publications as *ABC News, The Atlantic, BBC News, The Daily Beast, The Daily Mail, Elle, Feministe, The Good Men Project, Good Vibrations, The Guardian, Gurl, The Huffington Post, The Independent, Marie Claire, Metro, New Idea, New Scientist, Psychology Today, Salon, Scientific American, The Sun, The Telegraph,* and *XOJane.*

A long list of articles, with links to their Internet versions where applicable, is published on this collective:

http://juliesondradecker.com/?page_id=2091

Asexuality-Related Professional Video Media

Quite a few television programs, talk shows, and documentary series have been made about asexuality. Asexual guests have been featured on *20/20, Montel Williams, CNN, The Morning Show, HuffPost Live, MTV, The View,* and more, plus a full-length documentary titled *(A)sexual* was produced by Arts Engine (director: Angela Tucker) in 2011. The documentary is available on Netflix and can be followed at http://asexualthemovie.com/. More asexuality-related professional video media pieces are collected here:

http://juliesondradecker.com/?page_id=2080

(Note that some of these shows and TV spots are more sensationalistic than others.)

Asexuality-Related Audio Interviews, Presentations, and Podcasts

- **Asex 101:**
  David Jay's three-part lecture.
  Audio: http://media.libsyn.com/media/asexualunderground/asex101.mp3
  PowerPoint: http://www.asexuality.org/resources/asex_101.ppt

- **How Asexuality Works:**
  Stuff You Should Know did a half-hour feature on asexuality.
  Audio: http://castroller.com/Podcasts/StuffYouShould/3009746

- **Radio Netherlands Worldwide:**
  Interview of Nathan Royle.
  Audio:http://content1a.omroep.nl/a9dcc715074b50a02152d492a8b5792a/
  4fa20c31/rnw/smac/cms/tswi_the___a___word_20090829_44_1kHz.mp3

- **The Authority Smashing! Hour:**
  David Jay and swankivy Interview by host Zeno.
  Audio: http://www.blogtalkradio.com/tash/2010/09/09/the-authority-smashing-hour
  Transcript: https://docs.google.com/document/pub?id=1g1FXBTadt-tHxdF3-jMi0UkOGTkJ8HxadQTtiXMNh-o0

- **Savage Love:**
  David Jay appears on Dan Savage's show.
  Audio: http://www.thestranger.com/SavageLovePodcast/archives/2011/07/12/savage-love-episode-247
  Transcript: http://nextstepcake.tumblr.com/post/7568069160/transcript-david-jay-interviewed-on-savage-love

- **To the best of our KNOWLEDGE:**
  David Jay gives an interview to Anne Strainchamps.
  Audio: http://ttbook.org/book/redefining-romance-david-jay-asexuality
  Transcript: http://ttbook.org/book/transcript/transcript-redefining-romance-david-jay-asexuality

- **CBC's Q:**
  Modern Love segment interviews David Jay.
  Audio: http://www.cbc.ca/q/blog/2012/01/19/asexual-activist-david-jay-on-q/

- **Sex Out Loud:**
  David Jay on asexuality, interviewed by Tristan Taormino.
  Audio: http://www.voiceamerica.com/episode/66453/david-jay-on-asexuality

- **WNPR: Colin McEnroe:**
  Colin McEnroe interviews David Jay, Kathy Way, Tony Bogaert, and Julie Decker on "How Asexuals View the World."
  http://wnpr.drupal.publicbroadcasting.net/post/how-asexuals-view-world

- **A Life:**
  "*A Life* is a weekly podcast about asexuality and asexuals. The show is open to topic suggestions or listener questions and is always welcoming towards people who want to come on as a guest or perhaps even a regular panelist."
  http://alifepodcast.wordpress.com/

- **Unscrewed and Illuminated:**
  "A podcast about asexuality, all the issues that surround asexuality and the lives of asexuals. Prone to hilarious random tangents into a wide variety of topics."
  http://unscrewedandilluminated.galileoace.com/

Internet Videos and Channels on Asexuality

- **The Asexuality Top 10:** Channel swankivy
  "This is my top ten countdown about the misconceptions concerning asexuality. It begins with an introduction on what asexuality is, continues down a top ten list of most commonly suggested reasons for my lack of interest in sex and my refutations of them, and a follow-up honorable mentions catch-all video."
  http://www.youtube.com/playlist?list=PLF64276F6C84C6CBE

- **Letters to an Asexual:** Channel swankivy
  "I read the letters I get regarding asexuality and answer questions, tackle criticisms, and rebut nastiness as needed."
  http://www.youtube.com/playlist?list=PL70DADE9AE5417828

- **Hot Pieces of Ace:** Channel HotPiecesofAce
  "*Hot Pieces of Ace* is a YouTube collab channel designed to help the asexual community in any way imaginable . . . that can be captured on film."
  http://www.youtube.com/user/HotPiecesofAce

- **NO SEX?! - ASEXUALITY:** Channel lacigreen
  "This video covers the basic questions asked about an asexual orientation."
  http://www.youtube.com/watch?v=77o83_U8O5o

- **Asexual Bingo:** Channel swankivy
  "Sometimes silly, sometimes serious, and always with lots of bad language and inappropriate graphics, here is a capsule view of the kinds of comments I get on my YouTube videos and through other channels regarding asexuality."
  http://www.youtube.com/watch?v=ncoHJo5128Q

- **Asexuality:** Channel republicofsandals
  "A collection of videos on Asexuality."
  http://www.youtube.com/playlist?list=PL732D7335BEAA40DB

- **ACESOMNIACS:** Channel ACESOMNIACS
  "Vlogs about asexuality topics by some random AVENites."
  http://www.youtube.com/user/ACESOMNIACS

- **Shit People Say to Asexuals:** Channel swankivy
  A collection of what people say to asexual people: collaborative project of sixteen asexual people.
  http://www.youtube.com/watch?v=WBabpK_nvs0

- **Everything's A-Okay:** Channel AOkayVideo
  "Whoever you may be, know that you're not alone. You are a-okay just the way you are. Don't ever forget that."
  http://www.youtube.com/user/AOkayVideo

- **Queer As Cat:** Channel QueerAsCat
  "This channel will be home to my video blogs regarding asexuality, pan-romanticism, biromanticism, gender neutrality and more."
  http://www.youtube.com/user/QueerAsCat

- **Ace Ideas:** Channel UCWne6-e7QHSu74eM2hh7NkA
  "We are a diverse group of asexuals here to share our knowledge, experiences, passions, hobbies, and stories surrounding our asexuality."
  http://www.youtube.com/channel/UCWne6-e7QHSu74eM2hh7NkA

More channels and videos about asexuality are collected here:
http://juliesondradecker.com/?page_id=2083

Asexuality-Related Blogs

There are hundreds of asexuality-related blogs and blogs by asexual people on the Internet. They move, close, and get abandoned too frequently to list reliably here, but they are sometimes the best places to understand what asexual people are going through, to give and receive advice, and to connect to others.

AVEN has a partial list of blogs here:
http://www.asexuality.org/wiki/index.php?title=Asexual_Sites

A fairly long list of asexuality-related blogs is here:
http://juliesondradecker.com/?page_id=2077

"Asexual Perspectives" Contributors

ANDREW HINDERLITER
Asexual Explorations
http://asexystuff.blogspot.com

AUDACIOUS ACE
Asexuality Unabashed
http://audaciousace.blogspot.
com

AYDAN SELBY
Confessions of an Ist
http://greenchestnuts.
blogspot.com
The Asexual Agenda
(Contributor)
http://asexualagenda.
wordpress.com

DALLAS BRYSON
The Asexual Sexologist
http://asexualsexologist.word-
press.com

FIISH
http://apollyptica.tumblr.com

ILY
Asexy Beast
http://theonepercentclub.
blogspot.com

JO QUALMANN
A Life Unexamined
http://alifeunexamined.word-
press.com/

KAZ
Kaz's Scribblings
http://kaz.dreamwidth.org/

LAURA
Notes of an Asexual Muslim
http://ace-muslim.tumblr.com/

M. LECLERC
HYPOMNEMATA
http://hypomnemata.me

MARY KAME GINOZA
Next Step: Cake
http://nextstepcake.wordpress.
com

QUEENIE
Project Awesome
http://queenieofaces.tumblr.com
The Asexual Agenda
(Contributor)
http://asexualagenda.
wordpress.com

REBECCA
seiji has many socks.
http://4seiji.tumblr.com

SCIATRIX
Writing From Factor X
http://writingfromfactorx.word-
press.com
The Asexual Agenda
(Contributor)
http://asexualagenda.
wordpress.com

TOM
Asexuality Archive
http://www.asexualityarchive.
com

TRISTAN MILLER
The Asexual Agenda (Owner)
http://asexualagenda.
wordpress.com/
Skeptic's Play
http://skepticsplay.blogspot.com

Bibliography

ABC 20/20. (2006, March 27). *Sex Therapist Q&A*. Retrieved May 2, 2012, from ABC News: http://abcnews.go.com/2020/story?id=1759769&page=1#. T6DVlFJWJxV

American Psychiatric Association. (2000). *Diagnostic and Statistical Manual of Mental Disorders (4th ed.)*. Washington DC: American Psychiatric Association.

American Psychiatric Association. (2013). *Diagnostic and Statistical Manual of Mental Disorders (5th ed.)*. Arlington, VA: American Psychiatric Publishing.

Asexual Awareness Week. (2011, October 24). *Asexual Community Census 2011*. Retrieved October 24, 2011, from Asexual Awareness Week: http://facebook. com/notes/asexual-awareness-week/results-of-the-asexual-community-census-2011/208581089214485

Asexual Sexologist. (2012, February). *Asexuality Curriculum*. Retrieved May 9, 2012, from Asexual Sexologist: http://asexualsexologist.wordpress.com/ curriculum/

Asexual Visibility and Education Network. (2008). *About Asexuality: Overview*. Retrieved May 3, 2012, from Asexual Visibility and Education Network: http://www.asexuality.org/home/overview.html

Asexuality. (2002, December 11). Retrieved August 23, 2013, from Wikipedia: http://en.wikipedia.org/wiki/Asexuality

Banner, L., Whipple, B., & Graziottin, A. (2006). Sexual Aversion Disorders in Women. In H. Porst, & J. Buvat, *ISSM (International Society of Sexual Medicine) Standard Committee Book, Standard practice in Sexual Medicine* (pp. 320–324). Oxford: Blackwell.

Bogaert, A. (2013, September 9). The Colin McEnroe Show. (C. McEnroe, Interviewer)

Bogaert, A. F. (2004). "Asexuality: Prevalence and Associated Factors in a National Probability Sample". *Journal of Sex Research*, pp. 279–287.

Brotto, L., & Yule, M. (2011, August). Physiological and Subjective Sexual Arousal in Self-Identified Asexual Women. *Archives of Sexual Behavior*, pp. 699–712.

Brotto, L., Knudson, G., Inskip, J., Rhodes, K., & Erskine, Y. (2010, June). Asexuality: a Mixed-Methods Approach. *Archives of Sexual Behavior*, p. 599.

Cormier-Otaño, O. (2011, October 24). Spotlight on Asexuality Studies. *Doing Without: a Therapist's Findings*. Coventry, United Kingdom.

Diamond, L. M. (2008). *Sexual Fluidity: Understanding Women's Love and Desire*. Harvard University Press.

Emens, E. F. (2014). Compulsory Sexuality. *Stanford Law Review, 66.*

Gilmour, L. P., & Schalomon, M. (2012). Sexuality in a Community Based Sample of Adults with Autism Spectrum Disorder. *Research in Autism Spectrum Disorders,* pp. 313–318.

Girshick, L. B. (2008). *Transgender Voices: Beyond Women and Men.* UPNE.

Hope, A. (2012, May 16). *Does Asexuality Fall Under the Queer Umbrella?* Retrieved March 30, 2013, from Huffington Post: http://www.huffingtonpost.com/allison-hope/asexuality-queer-umbrella_b_1521191.html

Intersex Society of North America. (2008). *Intersex Conditions.* Retrieved May 10, 2012, from Intersex Society of North America: http://www.isna.org/faq/conditions

Kim, E. (2011). Asexuality in disability narratives. *Sexualities,* 479-493.

Kinsey, A. C. (1948). *Sexual Behavior in the Human Male.* Bloomington: W.B. Saunders Company.

Lasciel. (2011, August 10). *Was I Fired Because of My Asexuality?* Retrieved March 13, 2013, from Asexual Cupcake: http://thecupcakeace.wordpress.com/2011/08/10/was-i-fired-because-of-my-asexuality/

MacInnis, C. C., & Hodson, G. (2012, September 1). Intergroup Bias Toward "Group X": Evidence of Prejudice, Dehumanization, Avoidance, and Discrimination against Asexuals. *Group Processes & Intergroup Relations,* pp. 725–743.

McClintock, M. K., & Herdt, G. (1996, December). Rethinking Puberty: The Development of Sexual Attraction. *Current Directions in Psychological Science,* pp. 178-183.

McIntosh, P. (1989, July). White Privilege: Unpacking the Invisible Knapsack. *Peace and Freedom,* pp. 10–12.

Medical Letter on Drugs and Therapeutics. (1992, August 7). Drugs That Cause Sexual Dysfunction: An Update. *Medical Letter on Drugs and Therapeutics,* pp. 73-78.

Miller, H. B., & Hunt, J. S. (2003). Female Sexual Dysfunction: Review of the Disorder and Evidence for Available Treatment Alternatives. *Journal of Pharmacy Practice,* pp. 200–208.

Minto, C. L., Crouch, N. S., Conway, G. S., & Creighton, S. M. (2005). XY Females: Revisiting the Diagnosis. *BJOG: an International Journal of Obstetrics and Gynaecology,* pp. 1407–1410.

Phillips, N. A. (2000, July 1). Female Sexual Dysfunction: Evaluation and Treatment. *American Family Physician,* pp. 127–136.

Prause, N., & Graham, C. A. (2007). Asexuality: Classification and Clarification. *Archives of Sexual Behavior,* pp. 341–56.

Regan, P. C. (1999). Hormonal Correlates and Causes of Sexual Desire: A Review. *The Canadian Journal of Human Sexuality*, 1–16.

Rosenbury, L. A., & Rothman, J. E. (2010). Sex In and Out of Intimacy. *Emory Law Journal*, 809–868.

Savage, D. (2009, September 10). *The Truth About Asexuality: It's Just as Confusing as All of the Other Ones*. Retrieved June 8, 2011, from Savage Love: http://thecoast.ca/halifax/the-truth-about-asexuality/Content?oid=1263048

Scherrer, K. (2008). Coming to an Asexual Identity: Negotiating Identity, Negotiating Desire. *Sexualities*, pp. 621–641.

Scherrer, K. S. (2009). Asexual Relationships: What Does Asexuality Have to Do with Polyamory? In M. Barker, & D. Langdridge, *Understanding Non-Monogamies* (pp. 154-160). New York: Routledge.

Steketee, G., & Foa, E. B. (1987). Rape victims: Post-Traumatic Stress Responses and Their Treatment: A Review of the Literature. *Journal of Anxiety Disorders*, 69–86.

Tomchek, S. D., & Dunn, W. (2007). Sensory Processing in Children With and Without Autism: A Comparative Study Using the Short Sensory Profile. *American Journal of Occupational Therapy*, 190–200.

Tucker, A. (Director). (2011). *(A)sexual* [Motion Picture].

Yang, M. L., Fullwood, E., Goldstein, J., & Mink, J. W. (2005). Masturbation in Infancy and Early Childhood Presenting as a Movement Disorder: 12 Cases and a Review of the Literature. *Pediatrics*, 1427–1432.

Yoshino, K. (2000). The Epistemic Contract of Bisexual Erasure. *Stanford Law Review*, 353–461.

Yule, M. A., Brotto, L. A., & Gorzalka, B. B. (2013, March 7). Mental Health and Interpersonal Functioning in Self-Identified Asexual Men and Women. *Psychology & Sexuality*.

INDEX

House, M.D. (television show), 82
Housing discrimination, 58–59
Huge (television show), 81
Hulme, Keri, 81
Humor, appreciation of sexual, 125–126
Hypoactive sexual desire disorder, 59, 97, 129

Ignition Zero (Heimpel), 81
Illnesses, asexual people with, 79–80
Ily, 109, 124, 199
Internet-based asexual communities, 67, 187–190
Internet videos, 197
Intersex individuals, 10
Interviews, on asexuality, 194
Intimate activity. *See* Sexual activity
Intimate closeness, 32–33
Invisibility, 62–63, 66–67
Islam, 111

Jay, David, xiii, 191, 195, 196
Jokes
        within asexual communities, 82–84
        with sexual references, appreciation of, 125–126
Judaism, 111

Kaz, 12, 181, 199
Kink, 33–35
Kinsey Scale, 84

Lagerfeld, Karl, 81
"Late bloomers," 151–152
Latina/Latino people, 73
Laura, *Notes of an Asexual Muslim*, 7, 199
LeClerc, M., 11, 60, 104, 110, 119, 199
Lesbian asexual, 20
LGBT people
        asexual communities and, 75
        discussing their issues, 51–52

NOTES

NOTES

NOTES

NOTES

NOTES

NOTES

NOTES